Integrating Art Therapy and Yoga Therapy

Integrating Art Therapy and Yoga Therapy

Yoga, Art, and the Use of Intention

Karen Gibbons

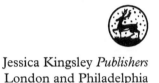

Jessica Kingsley *Publishers*
London and Philadelphia

First published in 2015
by Jessica Kingsley Publishers
73 Collier Street
London N1 9BE, UK
and
400 Market Street, Suite 400
Philadelphia, PA 19106, USA

www.jkp.com

Library of Congress Cataloging in Publication Data
A CIP catalog record for this book is available from the Library of Congress

British Library Cataloguing in Publication Data
A CIP catalogue record for this book is available from the British Library

ISBN 978 1 84905 782 0
eISBN 978 1 78450 023 8

Printed and bound in Great Britain

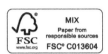

I dedicate this book with loving gratitude to all my teachers, including my amazing family, who impart valuable lessons daily.

ACKNOWLEDGMENTS

This book would not have been possible without the support of friends and family too numerous to name, as well as many wonderful teachers through the years who have made the process of acquiring my multi-disciplinary education an amazing journey.

In an attempt to name a cherished few, I would like to send deep gratitude to Mary Flinn, Joyce Cossett and the amazing Energy Center community who gently set me on "the path." Next, I would like to acknowledge chairman of the art therapy department at the School of Visual Arts, Deborah Farber, and the entire faculty, who helped me in a thousand ways to hone my skills and appreciate my calling. As the journey continues, Lisa Furman deserves a special mention as an exemplary supervisor and guiding light. Finally, I am so grateful to Joseph and Lillian LePage and all of the open-hearted teachers at Integrative Yoga Therapy, whose beautiful spirits inspired and informed me in my quest to become a yoga therapist.

CONTENTS

NOTES ON TEXT

Disclaimer

The recommendations here are for educational purposes only. Participation should be attempted only with suitable experience and supervision. Please consult a physician before beginning any yoga or exercise program and seek medical attention if you experience pain or other physical concerns. Neither the publishers nor author will accept any responsibly for any ill effects resulting from the use or misuse of the information contained in this book.

Notes on Chapters 6 through 9

These chapters give detailed instructions for performing the mudras, meditation, yoga poses and art directives shown in the Practice Chart for Intention Centered Yoga and Art (Table 5.1, pages 55–66). Although the elements are common knowledge to those in the respective fields of yoga and art therapy, I would like to acknowledge the following sources, which offer helpful compilations of pertinent information.

Mudras are ancient and commonly acknowledged in the Hatha yoga tradition. My knowledge of mudras and their use primarily comes from my education with Joseph and Lillian LePage during my integrative yoga training and from their recent book, *Mudras for Healing and Transformation*.[1]

---

1   J. LePage and L. LePage (2013) *Mudras for Healing and Transformation*. Sebastopol: Integrative Yoga Therapy.

There are many commonly acknowledged yoga poses. I would like to note that my knowledge of the poses and their descriptions comes from my training, originally at the Energy Center in Brooklyn, NY with Mary Flinn and Joyce Cossett. I would like to urge those wishing to learn teaching techniques to seek out a Yoga Alliance certified yoga teacher training program. For descriptions and advice, excellent print and online sources exist. I trust the information in B. K. S. Iyengar's *Light on Yoga*[2] and *Yoga Journal's* extensive online resources (www.yogajournal.com).

Art therapists are experts at devising art directives to suit the needs of their clients. I received my training at the School of Visual Arts in NYC. I draw from my own store of knowledge for these directives but also consult other sources for new ideas or to remember old standards. Excellent online sources include Shelly Klammer's list of *100 Art Therapy Exercises*,[3] Carol McCullough-Dieter's *Find Art Directives*[4] and Deborah R. Corrington's blog *Sharing Directives.*[5]

2   B. K. S. Iyengar (1995) *Light On Yoga*. New York: Schocken Books (original work published in 1966).

3   Klammer, S. (2014) *100 Art Therapy Exercises – The Updated List!* Expressive Art Workshops. Accessed on December 3, 2014 at www.expressiveartworkshops. com/expressive-artists/100-art-therapy-exercises.

4   McCullough-Dieter, C. (2010) *Find Art Directives*. Accessed on December 3, 2014 at http://findartdirectives.com/therapist_login.php.

5   Corrington, D. R. (2014) *Art Therapy: Sharing Directives*. Art Therapy Directives: Blogspot. Accessed on December 3, 2014 at http://arttherapydirectives.blogspot. com/2012/07/boundary-drawings.html.

PREFACE
My story

Once upon a time, I was an artist-mother-couch potato living with my young family. When I began to practice yoga in earnest I had three small children. My twins were seven and my younger son was four years old. I began to drag myself up the single flight of stairs to my neighbor's loft, where she would teach yoga classes once a week. I would practice my heart out for an hour and a half, feeling very unfit. After all, my main source of exercise was running after children, all of whom had emerged from high-risk pregnancies confined to bed rest. No wonder my muscles were quivering in those early poses. I would leave each class feeling triumphant. I was thrilled with the "high" I got from doing yoga, and with the simple fact that I had made it through the class. Afterwards, sore muscles would be with me for days and I would say to myself, "I'm never doing that again!" I would keep saying it until the day before the class when I'd finally be able to move properly without pain. Then my thinking would shift and I'd say, "Let's see what the teacher is doing this time!"

Over time, I began to love the way I felt after yoga. That feeling began to last longer and, at the same time, the sore muscles would fade more quickly. I was getting stronger in many ways. I became a less reactive parent. I began to understand how to make space for myself. I had always made time, however little, for making art. While it did not create more time, practicing yoga was giving me insight into myself that helped my art get to the point more quickly. I began to see that the quiet place I could find by messing with art materials was the same place I sought in my yoga practice. Cultivating both an art practice and a yoga practice was improving my mental health. Everyday challenges that previously left me anxious and depressed were now faced with good humor. I noticed ease in social situations that had never existed before.

One day, my teacher asked me if I would consider doing the teacher training at the local yoga studio where she was teaching. I laughed out loud! I said, "Don't be silly, I've barely practiced yoga." I truly had no thought of doing anything more than getting my act together. Yoga had revived my energy and revealed a way to get a handle on my life. From the time my twins were born I had been running a ragged marathon. Finally, I was choosing when to sprint and when to slow to a walk. A few weeks later, my teacher asked me again. She said, "You should apply to the teacher training program." And suddenly, like a switch had been flipped, I said, "OK, what do I have to do?" I applied, was accepted, and began the three-month program all in a span of about three weeks. I really had no idea what I was getting into, but I jumped in with both feet. I wanted to deepen my practice, which I certainly did. Everything was new. I had never even heard of a sutra or a mudra or much of anything else we were learning. And the practice schedule was intense. My mind and my body were opening and absorbing and I was truly transformed. I am as proud of that hard-earned 200-hour yoga training as I am of anything I have done.

Around the same time my teacher was suggesting a yoga teacher training, I had been toying with the idea of studying art therapy. I had been teaching preschool art classes for several years. I loved seeing children discover their creative selves and witnessing their work blossom into unique forms of self-expression. I was also enjoying many fabulous art experiments with my own children, observing powerful moments of self-possession, growth and insight. This was also around the time that my older son received a diagnosis of Asperger's syndrome, a mild form of autism. The diagnosis was a confirmation of what we already knew; this was a child who had his own way of experiencing the world. His uniqueness created challenges for him, of course, but also challenged us as a family. And as I'm sure you can imagine, the other two children had their unique challenges to contribute as well. I had begun to realize that the gifts that allowed me to negotiate my family and my preschoolers with grace and enthusiasm could be honed and expanded. I attended an open house for a master's level art therapy program and a light bulb went off. Art therapy beautifully married my skills. I knew why I made art, but sometimes wondered why I longed to connect with the viewer. I began to understand that it is because when a piece of art is successful, a viewer might be able to vicariously "get" that transcendent, indescribable, healing place that the artist experienced in its creation. I would like everyone to experience this flow state (Kolter 2014). I realized that in practicing art therapy I would get to help others to find that healing place in a way that could work for them. The master's program seemed perfect for me; and I was drawn, perhaps guided, toward two intense years of grad school.

I had finished my yoga training in 2003, thinking right up until the graduation ceremony that I had no intention of teaching. During the ceremony, reflecting on how much had changed for me, I suddenly realized that I had to share my transforming experience of yoga. I began to teach right away. I continued to study and expand my knowledge. When I began art therapy studies, I recognized that psychology, yoga philosophy, and art were all one endeavor for me. My master's thesis was on yoga and art therapy with mentally ill and chemically addicted patients in outpatient rehabilitation. The study and practice of integrating these threads continues to be compelling and fascinating. Combining my passion for making art with my devotion to the yogic model of wellness was quite natural. It has become my life, and serves me well as a cohesive therapeutic modality (Gibbons 2013).

It has been some years now since that tender time when I completed my initial yoga training and embarked on this new career. And still, mind, body and spirit are always considered in my approach to therapy. The convergence of learning that allowed me to blend my practice of yoga and art therapy has led me to continue my education, always supporting integration. I have gone on to study Integrative Yoga Therapy (IYT) with Joseph and Lillian LePage because their approach to yoga therapy is a holistic one. To quote from the IYT's *Yoga Toolbox for Teachers and Students*, "Yoga is an ancient science of health for the physical body and balance for the mind and emotions that provides the foundation for the spiritual journey whose destination is self knowledge" (LePage and LePage 2005, p.2).

Similarly, art making is a holistic activity. The American Art Therapy Association (ATTA) says on their website notes that the use of art therapy blossomed as practitioners recognized that:

> The creative process of art making enhanced recovery, health and wellness. As a result, the profession of art therapy grew into an effective and important method of communication, assessment, and treatment with children and adults in a variety of settings. (AATA 2014)

The confluence of art therapy and yoga in my life has allowed me to dip my toes into the stream of awareness and self-knowledge. I wish to offer these tools to those who need help. Throughout my career I have tried the combination in various ways, sometimes focusing on yoga and bringing in art making or often blending yoga techniques, meditation and mindfulness with art therapy. In my experience, the success of combining art therapy with yoga depends on the integration of intention. I have witnessed beautiful, magical moments where clients seamlessly internalize their intention in the course of a single session. I have come to recognize that positive results are achieved when the practice remains simple and cohesive. Illuminating the process involved in creating the Intention Centered Yoga and Art Therapy Method is the aim of this book.

INTRODUCTION

Art therapy and yoga fit well together as an integrative modality not only because of the many attributes they have in common, but also because the complementary aspects of the two disciplines support the ultimate goal of both yoga and art therapy: generating healing and positive change. Yoga is traditionally practiced to achieve a calm clarity from which to transform the self and find inner peace (Kraftsow 1999). Art therapy uses the power of creative self-expression to promote healing and well-being (Malchiodi 1998). Understanding the similarities and differences between the two practices will help to create a program that can weave their strengths into an effective therapeutic approach.

This book is directed at mental health clinicians in the field of art therapy who wish to integrate yoga into their practice. The system recommended here is also suitable for yoga therapists wishing to add art techniques to their practice. Yoga teachers can support their student's well-being by using yoga and art techniques. In fact, anyone can use the Practice Chart for Intention Centered Yoga and Art (Table 5.1, pages 55–66) to address common concerns and create a personal practice that blends the use of yoga and art.

Both yoga and art therapy are healing modalities by themselves, however, art therapists have training and focus to address clinical concerns such as trauma and serious mental illness that would not be appropriate for yoga teachers and yoga therapists to address without specialized training and accreditation. The use of the Intention Centered Yoga and Art Therapy Method by mental health professionals requires an added dimension of care. A professional melding modalities must be careful to remain within their scope of practice (Weintraub 2013). Seek supervision if there is a question around clinical competency. Be clear with your clients about your training. An art therapist should not offer yoga therapy without proper training and certification and yoga teachers and yoga therapists cannot offer art therapy without master's level credentials. Both professions can happily and ethically use techniques related to art and yoga as long as they maintain clear boundaries and awareness of legal guidelines around the use of touch in therapy (Furman 2013).

ATTRIBUTES YOGA AND ART HAVE IN COMMON

* Experience-based

* Guided by intention

* Promotes self-awareness

* Encourages flow state

* Activates the limbic brain

* Reduces stress

* Encourages observation rather than judgment

* Adaptive

* Encourages change and healing

Both yoga and art are experience-based rather than intellectually-based activities. A person's mind can convince them of many things, but the body and creative intuition express the truth of one's experience. Research has found that emotions may be stored in the body (Van der Kolk 1994). By doing yoga, a person can access deep emotions and then by creating art, one can find a means of expression on a fundamental level, perhaps avoiding rigid defense mechanisms.

Creating intention, or setting a clear direction or focus, is traditionally a way to keep the practice of yoga goal-oriented (Kraftsow 1999). Intention, for art therapists, is established routinely as they work with their clients to create therapeutic goals. One goal common to art therapy and yoga is the promotion of self-awareness. Self-awareness is present when a person develops insight into their behavior and improves their ability to make conscious choices. The ability to make conscious choices is a priority for a serious yogi, much as it is for a psychotherapy patient (Cope 2000).

In conjunction with the shared aim of finding insight, yoga and art therapy work so well together because both practicing yoga and making art can create a flow state. The flow state is similar to being "in the zone" while playing sports. In this state, the ego (along with its incessant judging) takes a break and allows the intuitive self to act. The wisdom of natural creativity is found in the process; connections are made, clarity is enhanced and new perspectives may be gained. Yoga and meditation instructors may encourage mindful behavior in order to consciously induce flow states (Kolter 2014; Willitts 2014). Peak moments of creativity are integrally connected with the ancient wisdom of the body and so can foster healing of the body, mind and spirit (Diaz 1999).

When people find themselves in a flow state their limbic brain is activated. As Kraftsow (1999) notes in *Yoga for Wellness*, the limbic system links "the conscious, intellectual functions of the brain and the unconscious, mechanical functions of the body" (p.303), which explains how emotional response is directly affected by physical sensations, bypassing the conscious mind completely (Goleman 1995). For example, when trauma occurs the stress response is activated and the body goes into fight or flight mode without making a conscious decision. Heart rate increases, respiration quickens and blood pressure goes up. The limbic system modulates the stress response during yoga practice, so that heart rate, respiration rate and blood pressure are reduced. When the physiological response to stress is reduced people experience less anxiety and improved mood (Harvard Mental Health Newsletter 2009). The kinesthetic activity of making art has been shown to activate the limbic system as well. Soothing the limbic system with yoga may be preparation for the brain to be ready to move in to the more complex demands of art making (Hass-Cohen 2008).

When stress is reduced and a state of flow is induced, then the suggestion to observe rather than judge is easier to implement. The lack of competition and judgment sets yoga practice apart from athletics and distinguishes engagement in art therapy from participating in an art class. When a person is encouraged to observe themselves, their behavior and their creative output without feeling judged or pushed to achieve, they are more likely to be open to change. The beauty of both yoga and art therapy is that non-judgment is continually cultivated.

All of the attributes mentioned here make the use of yoga and art therapy endlessly adaptive. The combined practice can target a wide range of needs. With care and mindful application yoga and art together can offer healing and growth to almost any population.

COMPLEMENTARY ASPECTS

	Yoga	Art therapy
Starting point	body	mind
Medium	breath	art materials
Goal	calming the fluctuations of the mind	creative self-expression
Completion	stillness	processing oriented
Orientation	spiritual awareness	self-awareness

In celebration of the remarkable commonalities yoga and art therapy possess, this book intends to help practitioners develop a skillful plan for marrying the two approaches. As in any marriage, it is also important to enjoy the complementary aspects of the pairing. Clients can experience each session in a variety of ways because of the many ways that yoga and art can be received. In a combined practice, the verbal intention stated at the beginning has many opportunities to affect the client as the session progresses. Therapy is never a one-size-fits-all experience. Different people can hold the same experience in different ways. Clients bring their fears, preconceptions and resistances into the room each time. The specific elements chosen for use in each session (mudra, yoga pose, art directive) are carefully selected to reinforce the treatment goal expressed in the intention. Some people may find that yoga practices guided by the breath connect them with observations that are important to them, while others may find that art materials are ideal vehicles for similar connections. At other times, every aspect of the session might present a client with opportunities for improving self-awareness.

Self-awareness is generally thought of as "insight" in a psychotherapeutic context and therefore psychotherapy is considered non-spiritual. In yoga, spirituality is not associated with any specific religion or organized set of rituals or system of beliefs; instead it is an individual holistic journey where each person follows their interests, priorities and perspectives. The yogic orientation refers to the self-awareness gained in yoga practice as "spiritual." Misunderstanding arises when spirituality and religion are confused. As Gary Kraftsow explains (1999), traditionally yoga is "a comprehensive spiritual practice oriented toward purification…and realization" (p.3). Realization is the ability to look within and see the truth of our own being, known as samadhi, or pure consciousness. In samadhi, one is absorbed in the present moment and subject and object have no distinction. In sustained efforts of creativity, similar states are reached and, as in yoga, one begins to unite the self with the consciousness that inhabits everything (Franklin 2001).

The combined practice can promote the awareness that brings balance and strength to the whole person. When clients who participate in sessions combining yoga with art therapy are informed about the orientation of the session at the outset, they are able to make choices about how treatment will look for them. The advantage of being able to blend art therapy with a spiritual approach is that its holistic nature leaves room for clients to make their own distinctions and to initiate any religious content they wish (Furman 2013).

The goal of yoga, according to the *Yoga Sutras of Patanjali*, is to calm the fluctuations of the mind (Satchidananda 2012). With yoga practices, an individual or group can ground their bodies and quiet the mental distractions they bring to the session. Calming the mind and coming to stillness can be especially supportive of the art therapy process. At the beginning of a session, using the Intention Centered Yoga and Art Therapy Method, a verbal intention is established. Yoga mudras, meditation and poses bring the intention into the physical realm. Next, the art directive inspires creative expression related to the intention's focus. Finally, at the end there is verbal processing of the experiential events. There is a good chance that creative self-expression can flow as the session comes full circle. Clients leave having had the opportunity to grasp the intention in a holistic way, through mind, body and spirit.

This book will show how to successfully blend the benefits of yoga and art into a single therapeutic practice. The Practice Chart for Intention Centered Yoga and Art, the centerpiece for the method, can be found in Chapter 5, pages 55–66. It is a numbered guide for 32 sequenced practices. Each row of the chart outlines a new sequence that can be used personally by anyone, or have clinical applications for art therapists and yoga therapists.

Chapter 1

MODALITIES

Art therapy

Art therapy is a wonderful modality with application to almost any population, as is evident from the American Art Therapy Association's (2013) description:

> Art therapy is a mental health profession in which clients, facilitated by the art therapist, use art media, the creative process, and the resulting artwork to explore their feelings, reconcile emotional conflicts, foster self-awareness, manage behavior and addictions, develop social skills, improve reality orientation, reduce anxiety, and increase self-esteem. A goal in art therapy is to improve or restore a client's functioning and his or her sense of personal well-being. Art therapy practice requires knowledge of visual art (drawing, painting, sculpture, and other art forms) and the creative process. (p.1)

In the United States art therapy is a credentialed profession where the Art Therapy Credentials Board (ATCB 2014) sets national standards for ethical and competent practice. The practice may also be licensed by state regulating bodies to assure that art therapists are properly educated and experienced in working in the field of mental health and wellness.

Art therapists may be familiar with people observing the effects of their work and calling it "magic." This is because much of the therapeutic effects occur non-verbally and the client effortlessly accesses the unconscious (Wallace 1987). Art therapy stands alone as a mental health treatment in that it allows a person to access their

However, the greatest benefits derived from art making in a therapeutic setting are the result of the therapist creating relationships, applying their skills and considering the qualities of art materials and imagery in relation to various client groups. Art therapists are experts at matching benefits to needs.

Yoga

> Yoga was developed up to 5,000 years ago in India as a comprehensive system for well-being on all levels: physical, mental, emotional and spiritual. While Yoga is often equated with Hatha yoga, the well-known system of postures and breathing techniques, Hatha yoga is only a part of the overall discipline of Yoga. Today, many millions of people use various aspects of Yoga to help raise their quality of life in such diverse areas as fitness, stress relief, wellness, vitality, mental clarity, healing, peace of mind and spiritual growth. (Yoga Alliance 2014)

This is a beautiful description of yoga today, given by the Yoga Alliance, a non-profit professional organization in the United States, which registers yoga teachers after they have completed training at approved schools. Typically, the many styles of Hatha yoga have become established as an influential teacher develops a particular point of view and gains many followers who find their method effective. This is the case for Iyengar yoga, Ashtanga yoga, Kundalini yoga, Forest yoga, Anusara yoga, Integral yoga, Sivananda yoga and others. In this way, the various styles of Hatha yoga commonly practiced in the West might correspond to theoretical approaches in art therapy. Yoga has affinity with art therapy in that it is most efficacious in promoting wellness when the yoga instructor applies their knowledge and training with skill and sensitivity to the people and situations in which they are working (McCall 2007a).

The various styles of Hatha Yoga have in common that those who practice them find specific gains. According to *Yoga Journal*

(McCall 2007b), yoga improves flexibility, strength, circulation, oxygenation and may lower cholesterol. Documented emotional benefits include stress relief, reduced anxiety and improved self-control and concentration. Yoga studies have also shown increased serotonin levels, which may correlate with higher levels of happiness (Danhauer, Mihalko and Levine 2009).

Yoga therapy

The effects of yoga on the relaxation response and stress relief are well known (Benson and Klipper 2000). Similar to art making's ability to create a shift in brain functioning, yoga techniques cultivate activities that elicit calm and focus. In *Yoga Chikitsa*, Dr. Bhavanani (2013) states:

> Yoga is the science and art of quieting the subconscious mind, a way of life, skill in action, union of thought-word-deed, integration at all levels, the science of conscious evolution and the method to attain as well as the state of emotional and mental equanimity. (p.210)

While yoga is not usually thought of as a mental health treatment modality, it does have that role for some yoga therapists. One of the antecedents to modern yoga is Yoga Chikitsa, which can be translated from Sanskrit as yoga therapy. Traditionally, mental and physical health were equal components of the holistic health that the yoga practitioner would seek. Yoga Chikitsa is an individualized approach to personal health, which might include yoga poses, mudras and compliance with other yogic practices (Bhavanani 2013). The one-on-one approach with which yoga was practiced traditionally grew into varied approaches, which might be more familiar to Western yoga practitioners. Now it is more common to find classes where the instruction is not modified for individuals but instead the class members adjust to the teacher. Yoga therapists value the time-honored approach of working one on one, or if they lead a group they modify the practice for the individuals present with knowledge of their health status.

In more recent times, yoga therapy has become a profession with certification and accredited schools. The International Association of Yoga Therapists (IAYT) supports research and education and has worked since 1989 to establish yoga therapy as a healing profession. Specialized training at IAYT accredited schools is required for certification. The training prepares the practitioner to work with any health problem by treating the whole person using yoga techniques (IAYT 2014).

Mudras

Mudras are sometimes referred to as "yoga of the hands." Mudras are simply hand gestures that are used in all cultures. We all use hand gestures in our everyday lives and can acknowledge the power of a clenched fist, folded hands, or shoulders shrugged with palms facing up. The use of hand gestures culturally and religiously is universal. The effect of the gesture is felt in the body and may be so strong that it effectively communicates the feeling to others. The word "mudra" can be translated as "seal" or "attitude" (LePage and LePage 2013). In yoga, mudras have been used for health in the body, emotional balance and spiritual devotion for thousands of years. Here, we will focus on mudras that are traditionally recognized in Hatha yoga.

In the Hatha yoga tradition, mudras are understood as "energetic keys" to yoga's insights, which may be integrated into all levels of our being (LePage and LePage 2013). The shapes made with the fingers direct the incredible energy of the hands. The hands and fingers are capable of assuming many shapes, and thus mudras are a means of accessing many possibilities for potential healing. In Hatha yoga, the fingers are each associated with one of the five elements. The thumb is linked with the fire element. The index finger represents the air element. The middle finger is associated with ether or the space element. The ring finger corresponds to the earth element and finally, the pinky or little finger is linked with the water element. These elements are said to be the components of the universe and, therefore, by manipulating the fingers we can awaken "core qualities" in each gesture and begin to use the shapes as vehicles for uncovering our own inherent positive qualities (Menen 2010).

Mudras can be performed at any time. In fact, you might like to try Hakini mudra right now. Bring your hands to face one another in front of your navel. Then allow finger and thumb tips to meet, each meeting its same finger on the opposite hand. Hold the shape loosely open, as if your fingers were around a ball. Relax your shoulders and notice any shift in feeling. Many people will notice a sense of wholeness or integration. If you gave that mudra a try you might begin to notice that the more still and calm you become, the greater the effects of the mudra. This is why mudras are ideal to couple with meditation (LePage and LePage 2013).

Meditation

Everyone has an idea of what the word "meditation" means to him or her. Meditation is defined by Merriam-Webster (2014) as:

1. to engage in contemplation or reflection

2. to engage in mental exercise (as concentration on one's breathing or repetition of a mantra) for the purpose of reaching a heightened level of spiritual awareness.

Many forms of meditation offer techniques to transform the mind. Some popular forms of meditation are mindfulness, a Buddhist tradition, also known as Vipassana. Zazen is a Zen Buddhist term for seated meditation. Transcendental meditation involves the use of a mantra; while Kundalini meditation is often paired with kriyas, or actions, which are meant to carry energy upwards in a person's energetic body. Qi gong uses movement and breath to circulate and direct qi, or energy. Guided visualization is a technique whereby a person is guided to focus on an imaginary environment. Trancebased meditations are practices where awareness of one's self and environment are suppressed (Bair 2010).

Different styles are appropriate according to what you wish to achieve. Some meditators simply want to relax. Some would like time to contemplate their thoughts, others would like to slow down their thoughts and focus on being in the present. Some use meditation as a way to find clarity around emotional issues. The purpose of meditation in the context of this book is to aid in customizing a practice of yoga and art therapy for an individual or a group. This means that the focus will be on an intention that is used as a mantra, or repeated phrase. Seasoned meditators who have used a mantra will find this intention-centered approach familiar. The meditation recommended will couple a mudra and a specific intention. The mudra supports the energetic qualities of the chosen intention. The calm upright posture of meditation allows the mudra to help focus the energy of the body, and repeating the words of an intention helps to focus the mind. Meditation allows the person to lay the groundwork for integrating positive qualities into many levels of being.

Studies have shown that some of the benefits of meditation are reduced inflammation, lowered blood pressure, slower breathing rate, more relaxed muscles, greater immune system response and increased emotional balance (Corliss 2014). These findings have a wide application to physical and mental health. Calming the body, breath and mind, as we do in meditation, activates the parasympathetic nervous system, the part of the autonomic nervous system that maintains normal body/mind functions, slows heart rate and allows clear thinking (Cherry 2014). As in art making and yoga practices, the relaxation response occurs. This is the opposite of the fight or flight response called the sympathetic nervous system. The sympathetic nervous system tends to be stimulated by triggers in our daily lives that remind our body/mind of the real but no longer imminent dangers. When people were living with the ever-present danger of being eaten by a tiger, the body/

mind had to be able to respond quickly. At the first sign of mental or physical danger a cascade of biological reactions occur in order to mobilize the resources needed to deal with the threat. Now, we generally must avoid fighting and fleeing, even as the physiological conditions for this pattern are repeated over and over. The repetition of this body/mind scenario may lead to serious physical and mental health conditions. Meditation is a tool with documented success in calming the patterns of arousal that interfere with the ability to act as opposed to react (McDonald 2010; Stephens 2009).

Chapter 2

MIND, BODY, SPIRIT

Mind-body-spirit, holistic, New Age, yoga, spirituality – these notions are trending in the popular media. Therapy clients may be seeking holistic health solutions because of the increased cultural interest and media attention to such topics (Plante 2007). But some therapists may be wary. Therapy is not a place for trendiness. Additionally, art therapists sometimes struggle to build clear professional identities, in part, because clinical peers can sometimes be confused by art therapy as it combines art with therapy (Feen-Calligan 2012). Should another element be added? Why offer the holistic approach of Intention Centered Yoga and Art Therapy?

Art therapy – a holistic therapy

An art therapist inspires respect and develops a positive professional identity when that person has clarity about what they offer and confidence in its efficacy (Feen-Calligan 2005). Although art therapy has broad application and can be practiced with many different theoretical approaches, one might argue that art therapy is already a holistic practice; therefore, the desire to support and expand its effectiveness with complementary practices is natural and appropriate. For this book's purposes the terms "holistic" and "mind-body-spirit" are interchangeable. Mind-body-spirit, whatever your definition of each part might be, cannot actually be separated. The definition of holistic, according to Merriam-Webster's (2014) dictionary is: "relating to or concerned with wholes or with complete systems rather than with the analysis of, treatment

----

of, or dissection into parts." Perhaps the deeper desire beneath the hype of the healing trends is to move away from dissection, toward recognition of our wholeness. Art therapy does this very well (Malchiodi 1998).

Art therapy treatment begins with clinical skill, used to address the mental workings of the client, generally addressing concerns from a theoretical perspective. Art making is another indispensable tool for an art therapist. The body is used in the creation of art. With this activity, sensory integration occurs and the brain is activated in ways not possible with purely verbal therapy because of the complex interactive systems of the body. Finally, the therapist may enter the realm of the spirit in order to intuitively manage the synergistic process that occurs in any creative arts therapy (Lusebrink 2004; Ramm 2005).

In a holistic practice, intuition is considered the spirit's voice. Spirit might be referred to as the animating force, or life force, which exists in every living person, distinct from mind and body. Intuition is different from thought, which is generally accepted as a product of the mind. There may be intuitive clues noticed through felt sensations in the body, but it is not strictly a physical phenomenon either. Art therapists must use intuitive skills in their work because the creation of art itself depends on it; "a work of art begins with an intuition of the total form and the feelings embodied by it" (Julliard and Van Den Heuvel 1999, p.114). The intuition or spirit required to create a work of art was called "livingness" by Susanne Langer, an early seminal figure in art therapy, reflecting the fact that another component is needed in the creation of art, aside from the body and the mind. Langer even went on to challenge the idea that body and mind are separate: "Creating art demonstrates the unbroken continuum between what most people dichotomize as body and mind. Therein lies its potential for healing" (Julliard and Van Den Heuvel 1999, p.118).

In contrast, the field of psychology historically encouraged such a dichotomy in the interest of evidence-based science, denying the obvious: that a whole person is necessarily in possession of mind, body and spirit (Plante 2007). Although interest in partnering with alternative therapies has grown in recent years, there may be a lingering mistrust of holistic practices among those who have prioritized evidence-based practices. Evidence is important, and holistic practices are increasingly subjects of research, however, ideally research should be inspired by efficacy (O'Conner 2001).

While art therapists might alter their emphases to suit individual needs, they would not consider eliminating part of the process in order to become more oriented to a single aspect of a person. Because the practice of art therapy is a wonderful tool to address the whole person, it links well with other holistic methods. In the chapter on spirituality and art therapy in her book, *Ethics in Art Therapy*, Furman (2013) notes that many art therapists are drawn to alternative practices. She wisely points out that one should not confuse interest in complementary practices with training, and should take care to avoid dual relationships with clients. Art therapy treats the whole person with its "blend of intuitive and clinical skill, combined with a deep connection to the artistic and healing process" (Furman 2013, p.98). Implemented judiciously, the addition of other holistically oriented therapies to an art therapy practice can offer great potential for more complete healing (Plante 2007).

Who is yoga meant for?

There seems to be a yoga studio on every corner these days and it seems like they are full of young, flexible, fit people. What exactly is yoga and who is yoga for anyway?

Yoga in the West has grown exponentially in recent years and come to be associated mainly with the physical aspect of the practice. If you have spent time with the serious study of yoga then you know that the heart of the discipline has nothing to do with beautiful bodies. B. K. S. Iyengar (1995), in his influential book, *Light on Yoga* says, "Yoga is a timeless pragmatic science evolved over thousands of years dealing with the physical, moral, mental and spiritual well-being of man as a whole" (p.14). Iyengar goes on to translate the word yoga to mean union or yoke. In his view, the union referred to is describing the yoking of body, mind and soul. The yoga postures, known in Sanskrit as asana, are a small part of the self-discipline that will bring a person to the "real meaning of Yoga – a deliverance from contact with pain and sorrow" (Iyengar 1995, p.19).

Pain, whether physical or emotional, can be seen as misalignment. Iyengar's renowned teaching focused on alignment because physical alignment allows the life force to flow more freely through the body, which may in turn allow the mind to find optimal alignment. Donna Farhi (2005) calls the practice of yoga a "life practice. By life practice I mean an ongoing inquiry into how to be completely engaged and intimate with the wild force that runs through everything and is running through us, if we would but pause long enough to notice" (p.39). The knowledge that yoga is meant to enliven the whole person is helpful in understanding the use of yoga in the practices suggested in this book. The art and yoga techniques recommended in the coming pages are carefully aligned to have an engaging and enlivening effect on a person's life. The sequences are designed to be accessible enough for anyone to be able to pause and learn more about themselves.

As you can see, yoga is meant for everyone. However, the science of yoga is ancient and vast. There are a number of organizing principles that guide yoga philosophy. Students of yoga philosophy may learn about yoga's eight limbs, five koshas, 196 sutras and seven chakras in addition to pranayama (breathing practices), mantra, and the many paths of yoga. To complicate matters further, yoga studios offer many different styles of yoga. This complexity can be needlessly overwhelming. Probably all of the styles of yoga offered in studios in the West fall under the umbrella of Hatha yoga. Hatha refers to the path of yoga that concerns itself with physical yoga postures. Hatha practices also include attention to the mind, breath and meditation; cultivating a practice of balance. Hatha means sun (Ha) and moon

(Tha) and so refers to the balance of all natural forces. The Intention Centered Yoga and Art practices included in this book are meant to employ the principles of Hatha yoga in a simple and balanced manner, making them accessible to all (Lee 2014).

Factors to consider in making yoga approachable include timing, simplicity and ease of execution. In order to honor these considerations, only a few aspects of yoga will come into focus here. The components chosen are: intention, mudra, meditation and yoga poses. These elements will be explained in detail in the coming chapters. In an attempt to accommodate every level of practitioner, the language has been kept simple. Familiar words were chosen, like meditation and yoga pose. Yoga teachers will be familiar with the term asana, meaning posture, but even the neophyte knows what to expect from the term yoga pose. Please understand that if you have training and experience you may wish to use your expertize to modify the practices as you see fit, to best serve your clients.

Descriptive English titles were used to name the yoga poses rather than the traditional Sanskrit names. In the case of the mudras (hand gestures), their Sanskrit names were retained because there are no corresponding names in English. You may wish to educate those you work with about the terms and names for the various mudras, or you can simply refer to them as hand gestures and demonstrate or describe how to perform them rather than naming them.

All of the yoga techniques mentioned here encourage attention to the breath. Deep cleansing breaths are a way to increase focus and coordinate breathing, as well as to open and close the yoga practice. Many yoga practitioners are familiar with chanting the mantra "om" for this purpose. People new to yoga sometimes confuse chanting in Sanskrit with religious ritual, or are simply uncomfortable with the strangeness of the practice. In the interest of remaining clear about the secular nature of the yoga practice and to avoid misunderstanding, the deep cleansing breath has been substituted. If you and those you are working with wish to use the simple mantra (chant) of om please do so. Om is said to be the sound of universal consciousness, or the sound of the universe. It is lovely to notice that the sound of many voices becomes one sound, revealing the union that is yoga (Lee 2014).

Each step of the way you will make choices, deciding how best to use the material in this book to support the therapeutic relationship. The yoga journey was originally meant to become a way of life, undertaken with a guru, or teacher, who is "free of ego [and]…sees that he [the student] absorbs the teachings" (Iyengar 1995, p.28). The traditional yoga guru has a similar role to that of a therapist because an art therapist, yoga therapist and serious teacher of yoga all understand that learning and growth take place in relationship to each other. Yoga students were never meant to puzzle things out on their own. The same is true for clients of therapists who use the therapeutic relationship to develop trust and become attuned, affording the likelihood of security and growth (Gregson and Lane 2000).

Why add art making to the practice of yoga?

Yoga instructors who have a deep study of yoga philosophy could point to the many treatises on the subject and not find reference to art making. However, there is a strong correlation between yoga and creativity. Studies have shown yoga practitioners and meditators have brain patterns that correlate with those necessary for creativity. This includes the alpha waves that appear when the mind is relaxed and alert as well as measurements that correlate with novel ideas and insights (Davis 2012). The purpose of practicing yoga is to allow the effects to resonate in the rest of life. For yogi and art therapist Michael Franklin (2001), both practices are devotional because the person constantly witnesses creative effort with compassion. Franklin says, "These practices invite a rich, present-centered relationship of awareness to unfold…The wisdom of yoga philosophy helps… to understand the mystery of art and art therapy" (2001, p.97). Combining yoga with art making expands and enhances creativity and may enhance the expansion of personal insight as well. It appears that the two practices are mutually beneficial.

Combining modalities

When modalities are combined, ideally it is because they have both commonalities and complementary qualities. When the balance is right, the modalities can dovetail into a single approach. Art therapy and yoga have benefits and approaches in common because they both access healing non-verbally. The modalities differ in the tools they use for achieving these benefits. Art therapy uses hands-on involvement with art materials as the primary means to access novel ways for clients to learn more about themselves. Yoga uses attention to the physical body and the breath to access self-knowledge. Both modalities may promote stress relief, ability to focus, and work well to enable clients and students to shift habitual patterns.

The means used for achieving benefits in art therapy and yoga are complementary but have in common the ability to circumvent the verbally oriented emphasis of the thinking mind. Combining yoga and art therapy provides a holistic alternative to traditional talk therapy. For those in clinical practice it is exciting to have an approach to mental health treatment that is not primarily oriented toward psychopharmacology or verbal processing with the capability to consider the body as well as the mind. In fact, research on the neurobiology of resiliency indicates that an integrative approach to therapy using art therapy in conjunction with mindful techniques that utilize yoga and the breath can improve coping skills and help to balance dysregulation common for those affected by trauma and other psychosocial stressors (Hass-Cohen *et al.* 2014). As psychiatrist Bessel Van der Kolk (1996) explains it, "brain, body and mind are inextricably linked, and it is only for heuristic reasons that we can still speak of them as if they constitute separate entities. Alterations in any one of these three will intimately affect the other two" (p.216).

Action taken toward balance of the body, brain and mind is the healing impulse. According to Barbara Ganim (1999), "healing is an internal process. No person or thing can heal you. Only you can heal yourself. Healing restores balance and harmony to the body, mind and spirit" (p.44). The holistic healing available with a combined approach centers on establishing optimism, meaning and resolve – in short, consciously creating intention.

Chapter 3

- - - - - - - - - - - - - - -

INTENTION

The power of intention

Creating a yoga and art practice begins with forming an intention. What is an intention? Intention is a simple idea. Intention is defined as an aim or objective; an inspiration coupled with resolve. The resolve to produce a desired result pervades our every action. Suppose I am thirsty. Before I pick up a glass and turn on the tap for a glass of water I must form an intention. If I had to put words to it I would say, "I quench my thirst by drinking water." The power of intention is operating on a low level all the time. Imagine how well hydrated I would be if I upped the power level of that intention by repeating it aloud each time I was thirsty! The will allows us to make choices in which mind and body can work toward a common goal.

Psychologist Dr. Wayne Dyer maintains that we create our destiny by the innate power of intention (Dyer 2004). Intent is a force that exists in the universe. Dyer has studied the psychological, sociological and spiritual aspects of intention in order to discover how to harness the power that we use continually. The purpose of harnessing intention is to create the life you prefer to lead. Positive intention is formed from a combination of attention, self-respect and awareness.

Patanjali, in the ancient book of yogic wisdom, *The Yoga Sutras*, suggested a similar idea, referring to the power a person assumes when they are feeling inspired: "Dormant forces, faculties, and talents come alive" (Satchidananda 2003, p.14). In fact, yoga itself, sometimes defined as "the union of opposites," is achieved by intention (Sparrowe and Martinez 2008, p.10, first published 2002). When fully engaged in yoga practice one is simultaneously matter and essence, form and spirit – seeming opposites, fused in the act of intention. For this reason yoga practice, whether individual or group, commonly begins with the setting of an intention.

Intention is also linked to creativity. The formation of an intention is a creative act that holds the seed of self-expression (Dyer 2004). An artist begins any work of art with an intention. The powerful spark of intention is the inspiration behind art making. When artwork lacks inspiration it is no longer interesting to the viewer. The quality of intention and inspiration are important and mysterious ingredients in art. Art that is called "uninspired" is often work that is created by rote. The spirit that might enliven it is missing; it is form-heavy and lacking in essence.

The power of intention/inspiration in art therapy lies in the inherent power an art product holds for its creator. A work of art in art therapy is often created purely from inspired intention, rather than from developed skill, which has a greater possibility of being used habitually. Conscious intention to acknowledge our wounds makes it possible to release emotions and to truly heal. Making visual art is a way of becoming aware of feelings, thoughts and ideas, a way of constructing our world. Work begins with the body, the organically creative, physical self (Gibbons 2005). The yogic idea of "union of opposites" is precisely what guides artistic creation; thoughts and feelings take on a two- or three-dimensional form, simultaneous matter and spirit, when the artist's intention allows the mind to guide the artist's hand.

An artist consciously connects ideas with art materials to form full, clear expression. So too can intention be used consciously by connecting feelings with words to create phrases that fully express the intended result. In using intention with art or words, the key to success is the imagination. Imagination is the inner process where the outcome you wish for gives focus and energy to your willpower. Will alone is not very effective without imagination.

The process of consciously creating intention focuses the will and expands the possibilities for what can be accomplished. Dyer (2004) says, "Imagine myself to be and I shall be" (p.40). Aspirations are not achieved by strong will; the unlimited imagination is the fuel that allows the will to manifest intentions. Working with conscious intention is a way to train the imagination. The training involves imagining what it is you wish to attract more of in your life. An intention uses words and phrases to match the circumstances that you intend to have. The key to structuring an intention is to find a positive spin. If you allow your energy to go into complaining about what *is*, then you will actively participate in resistance. If you focus on gaining more of what you do want then you participate in the creation of the object of your desires. The positive approach of imagining and being open to the state of mind that you wish to cultivate holds creative power because it is rooted in self-respect. Self-respect honors your ability to take responsibility for yourself, and feeds self-confidence and self-esteem. Placing blame elsewhere, complaining, or deprecating the self are forms of resistance that block your ability to imagine yourself the way you would truly like to be. The power of intention lies in its power as a tool to imagine and create the outcome, the destiny that you intend.

How to create an intention

The purpose of creating an intention is to facilitate a shift from "concern" to "solution." Studies show that intention is a key factor in changing habitual behavior (DeBurijn *et al.* 2007). Habits are essentially well worn, reinforced neural pathways in the mind (Grohol 2005). Habits are changed by first bringing awareness to the negative aspects of the habit, something therapists are good at. Next, a person needs to establish a strong intention to change a habit. By carefully finding positive, present tense phrasing for the words that will be repeated one can focus the effects of the intention. Repetition builds new pathways. Better yet, with conscious application one can catch the old habits of mind and interrupt them with the intention for the solution (Downey 2010).

Intention is a framework to set up aspirations, aligning with the resources that make it possible. What makes an intention strong? It must be meaningful to the person creating it. Take the time to craft a phrase that resonates. In line with what Dyer (2004) calls "thinking from the end" (p.41), the intention is stated in the present tense. When you speak as if the end result, the way you would like things to be, already exists then you are directing energy and focus toward the actual accomplishment of the goal, as opposed to focusing on the obstacles that might prevent the goal from manifesting. Focus on obstacles just sets up thinking around limitations. At the same time, one must make the desired outcome both believable and reachable. Ideally, be able to feel and visualize the desired outcome. Beware of negativity! It may come naturally to phrase an intention around what is NOT wanted. Instead, focus on what you DO want. Also, avoid words that imply obligation such as "should," "always" or "never" or competition (even with yourself), such as "most," "best" or "more."

To state an intention aloud the speaker declares the goal to themselves as well as the world and the universe. Language that is empowering will support the effectiveness of the intention. Keep it short and sweet and it will be most effective. Also, it is convenient if the intention can be easily memorized and said by rote. Finally, for an intention to resonate with imagination, intuition and behavior it should feel clear, pure and energized.

Focus on the solution

The intention is the organizing element of this book's approach to combining yoga and art. You will see that the Practice Chart for Intention Centered Yoga and Art (Table 5.1) on pages 55–66 begins with a concern. The medical model that most Western mental health treatment is based on tends to be concern-focused. A client or patient comes with a list of symptoms or a concern-based label. It may be convenient to begin the process of planning a combined practice with the presenting "problem." However, as you gain experience with the elements of Intention Centered Yoga and Art you may find you naturally shift focus and begin to train the mind to look instead for what is needed. If your focus is on the solution you align with what is needed rather than what is lacking. Wayne Dyer (2004) says that one of the best ways to manifest your intention is to use imagination confidently to focus on the desired outcome, indifferent to doubt. Imagination is the basis for the creation of mudra, meditation, postures and art; to employ them all in the service of intention makes good sense.

STEPS TO CREATING AN INTENTION WITH CLIENTS

In the Practice Chart, (Table 5.1, pages 55–66) intentions are suggested and are meant to align with the recommended solutions to common concerns. Using the chart, you might find that the intention resonates as written, or you may wish to make alterations. The steps to create an intention with a client are as follows:

1. Speak about the concern and solution that you have selected. Does the solution "feel" right to the client? You may need to choose a different word or phrase that has the meaning and connotation that connects with the client. It may take some discussion for the client or group to respond to goal formation. Take time to identify what is needed accurately. Stay away from concrete solutions. The process of creating an intention is an intuitive one. Use the tools of intuition, free association, images, hunches and gut feelings.

2. After you have decided together what is needed, have the client describe what it would be like to have already

achieved this quality. Stay focused on the outcome. The more vividly the solution can be imagined, the closer it is to being achieved.

3. Ask the person to state the intention in the present tense as if it were already occurring. Encourage them to keep it short and to the point. Ideally, it should be easy to remember and can be repeated word for word right away. Have your client say it aloud so that they may take note of how it resonates. The right intention sits well in the mind and on the tongue. Groups can brainstorm a concept and you can restate it clearly in the present tense. Alternatively, you can offer the group an intention of your own devising and have them repeat it aloud, as you would for a brainstormed intention.

Chapter 4

THE INTENTION CENTERED YOGA AND ART THERAPY METHOD

There are many ways to go about blending the practices of yoga and art therapy. The aim of this book is to offer the combination as an accessible and easy-to-follow method, created around intention. The Practice Chart for Intention Centered Yoga and Art (Table 5.1), which you will find on pages 55–66, describes a structured way to deal with specific emotional issues.

Understanding the chart

On each row of the chart a sequence is proposed. The sequence is designed to have an effect on the whole person. First, a concern is identified and a possible solution is called to mind. An intention then invokes the desired outcome, speaking to the mind, body and spirit. On an energetic level, adopting a mudra reinforces the stated intention. Holding the mudra to meditate on the intention produces an inner focus and present moment awareness. The person literally embodies the qualities of the solution by assuming a yoga pose. Next, the act of creating art unites the physical and the intuitive, igniting the creative aspect of the person's psyche and bypassing the tendency to analyze and defend. Finally, the participant engages in

----

verbal processing to bring the effects of the various modalities to a conscious level. Coming full circle encourages all the elements to assimilate. This technique for integrating a person's physical, mental and intuitive capabilities can be a valuable tool for emotional regulation.

Personal practice

The Practice Chart for Intention Centered Yoga and Art (Table 5.1) works beautifully to guide personal practice. It can be used as a template for anyone who would like to combine art making with yoga and meditation. Use of the chart is meant to enable a person to find healing through self-awareness. The art techniques recommended are simple and the yoga mudras and poses are uncomplicated. Those willing to educate themselves about yoga and art can use the chart to enjoy the benefits of a specialized self-practice, whether or not they are guided by a therapist or yoga teacher.

Professional practice

The chart can also be used as a framework for therapeutically integrating yoga and art. An art therapist with an interest in yoga is likely to be eager to combine yoga with their established practice. Yoga teachers or yoga therapists sometimes have a creative flair and become intrigued with adding art making to the practice of yoga. The Practice Chart for Intention Centered Yoga and Art (Table 5.1) provides a guide for combining these modalities in a thoughtful manner. As discussed earlier, yoga and art techniques both have intrinsic positive effects on emotional balance. The techniques described here can be used to address concerns that are adjunctive to mental health diagnoses.

Sometimes people find the therapeutic process mysterious; indeed it can be powerful when everything works. A therapist knows that this happens because the therapeutic elements supporting the treatment goals identified for the client or group have been carefully balanced. When one therapeutically combines yoga and meditation with an art directive and concludes with cognitive processing, a potent protocol for restoring balance and fostering resiliency is activated (Hass-Cohen *et al.* 2014).

An illustration

It might be helpful to illustrate how the Practice Chart for Intention Centered Yoga and Art could be used. First, a clinician identifies a concern, and acknowledges a possible solution. For example, in Figure 4.1, an art therapist might find that the group that they are facilitating is restless and inattentive. The group's restlessness is impeding their clinical progress. By focusing on an ideal solution for the treatment concern, the clinician can adopt a non-judgmental stance and find the seed of an idea from which an intention may be created. In broad terms, the solution for restlessness is stillness. A simple statement in the present tense, which brings to mind the solution is created: "I am focused and still." Holding a hand gesture, or mudra, can then support the concept expressed in the intention.

Concern	Solution	Intention	Mudra for meditation	Yoga pose	Art directive
Restlessness	Stillness	"I am focused and still."	Kapota	Boat Pose	Create a CALMING COLOR LANDSCAPE using any art material.

Figure 4.1 Example from chart

Once the intention is established, the art therapist may ask the group to bring their hands into Kapota mudra. Kapota (where the hands come to prayer position and the fingers, thumbs and base of the palms stay together while the knuckles move away from each other) cultivates peace in the inner being. Combining mudra with intention creates a simple meditation. The therapist would then have the group hold Kapota mudra, close their eyes and meditate on the intention. After the brief meditation, a yoga pose is introduced; one with attributes that embody the solution to the original concern. Boat pose, a seated pose where the chest is lifted and the shins are held parallel to the ground, requires focus, strength and stillness. The participants hold the pose for five breaths.

At this point, the art therapist would quietly bring the group to a table to make art. The art directive continues to reinforce and demonstrate the qualities of focus and stillness put forth in the intention. The direction is to create a landscape in colors that each individual considers calming, using their preferred drawing material. The therapist would then end the session with verbal processing, which will allow the qualities of focus and stillness to be discussed on a conscious and personal level. The juxtaposition of intention, mudra, yoga pose and art directive creates a synergistic process. The thread of intention is woven through the session and the various ways its message is absorbed by the clients have a cumulative effect. The group might then end in a state of calm attentiveness.

The Practice Chart

I recognized the power of combining modalities from my personal practice. The chart was created because I wanted to organize my thoughts about how to structure classes, sessions and my personal practice around intention. In my experience, a more intuitive process produces more effective therapeutic value for my clients. Having sensible sequences readily at hand frees the practitioner to work intuitively and reduces time spent in thinking and analyzing. The sequences outlined in the chart are merely suggestions. The chart is a means of connecting the dots among related effects of yoga and art-making practices. There are many ways to connect the dots.

As readers become more experienced with yoga and art modalities they will be able to develop a repertoire of ideas of their own.

The Practice Chart for Intention Centered Yoga and Art begins with a concern, but in fact, a practitioner could begin at any point. The "solution" might be a starting point, and looking back at the concern would confirm whether or not the chart is serving your point of view. A practitioner could also begin with a pose in mind. The chart can then help determine if the pose would be appropriate and would clarify how it might work in conjunction with treatment goals. Maybe a person is attracted to a certain mudra; the chart can then help to align the mudra with an intention. The intentions make good starting points as well. The chart may suggest how to develop a practice around a chosen intention.

One important concept in the Practice Chart for Intention Centered Yoga and Art is the idea of "practice." To practice is a wonderful thing. It implies that a person is simply working with the elements at hand, on a journey of discovery. There is no goal of perfection, merely a process of carrying out an idea. In the course of practice one gains a sense of familiarity, playfulness and learning. In the yoga and the art-making practice offered here the aim is for people to learn more about themselves. The act of organizing thoughts into an intention, forming a mudra, meditating, holding a pose and then allowing those accumulated effects to blossom into the creation of art is a worthy practice of self-discovery.

Chapter 5

THE PRACTICE CHART FOR INTENTION CENTERED YOGA AND ART

Instructions for meditation and assuming mudras and yoga poses can be found in Chapters 6 through 9. Each component in the chart can be adapted for individual use. There are many more variations for mudras and yoga poses than could be included in the scope of this book. Yoga information is available from books (see Further Reading) and online sites as well as registered yoga instructors. Art directives should ideally be done with the materials specified. Art therapy practitioners might want to expand on the concepts suggested here, or devise their own directives to suit the intention.

Each sequence could be used for a personal practice, as an adjunct to clinical treatment, or as a group activity. The sequence could also serve as therapeutic "homework" for practitioners who work in that manner. The entire sequence will take from 15 minutes to an hour or more, depending on how long one remains in meditation, how long a yoga pose is held, and the intricacy of the art directive. Clinicians can adjust the timing according to their needs and preferences.

USING THE PRACTICE CHART FOR INTENTION CENTERED YOGA AND ART

1. Begin with an identified concern or simply find the healing concept you would like to work with from the "solution" column.

2. Be sure to have an area with enough space and privacy to complete the sequence.

3. Look over the art directive and gather the materials needed.

4. Read the intention and alter the wording, if necessary, to suit the person who will use it.

5. Pair the intention with the mudra for meditation. Sit quietly in a comfortable position with a straight spine. Eyes may be closed, or the gaze may be focused softly downward. Place the hands into the position of the mudra and take a deep breath in. Exhale and relax the shoulders. Repeat the intention three times aloud. Continue to repeat the intention silently, one time for each breath cycle. After ten breaths, say the intention aloud one time. Inhale deeply, exhale and release the mudra.

6. Assume the yoga pose. If the version of the pose pictured in the chart is not appropriate, please find a variation. Some will find a modified pose more comfortable and some will find a more challenging version of the pose to be more suitable. The pose should *always* be comfortable. Pain is to be avoided. If it is possible to breathe freely without holding the breath or laboring to breathe, then the pose can be held for five to ten breaths. If the pose is two-sided, then repeat the same number of breaths on the second side.

7. Quietly move to the art materials and follow the art directive.

8. Verbally discuss what it was like to create the artwork. Stay away from judgment words such as "like" and "good." Use observation words/phrases instead like, "I see..." or "I noticed..." If practicing alone, writing in a journal is recommended at this point.

Putting it all together

Just as there are many ways to put art materials together to create art, there are endless ways to blend the dynamic practices presented in this book. The chart provides a means for intention to guide the use of mudra, meditation, yoga poses and art making. The chart acts as an aid, but is not a substitute for developing knowledge of yoga and art combined. Your own practice of art and yoga supports the mindful style of professional practice that the Practice Chart for Intention Centered Yoga and Art (Table 5.1) is based on. Implementation of these practices will become natural as you discover how it best serves your clients. The yoga and art chart can streamline the process of putting together a practice; it can be a learning tool or a means of generating ideas. The structure is designed to create a flow of activity that supports the desired outcome. In the yoga and art chart specific mudras, poses and art ideas are suggestions. There is always a substitution that might work just as well, or be more appropriate for a given situation. As you become familiar with the elements and begin to use various combinations, you will find the right fit and create a useful practice for yourself and/or each person or group with whom you work.

The chart is also structured for convenience, beginning with a concern; typically a good starting point for a clinician who is trained to identify symptoms and assess for diagnosis. As a compassionate yoga and art facilitator you may prefer to work from the solution. Thinking about the solution supports a strengths-based practice that is empowering for the client and lends itself to creating intention. The intention is the pivotal element. In the yoga and art chart the choices of all the other elements relate to the qualities evoked in the intention. Creating an intention leads to identifying qualities that ideally will be included in each element. However, once you are familiar with the principals of all the aspects of a session, then any point of entry is a good one. When you have developed a working knowledge of mudras, yoga poses and art directives you will decide where your starting point will be.

For example, you might decide that a person would benefit from the steadiness that Mountain Pose has to offer. From there you can match up a mudra that has qualities of steadiness, such as the gesture of the little finger, Kanistha mudra, where the tips of the little fingers touch each other and the other fingers relax inward, toward the body. From there, an appropriate intention may be inspired by the emerging sensations, such as, "I exhale and feel my stability." Finally, one could devise a steadiness-promoting art intervention, perhaps inspired by the images evoked by the yoga posture, like drawing or sculpting a mountain. Allow me to elaborate on some pieces of the puzzle in the following chapters.

Table 5.1 Practice Chart for Intention Centered Yoga and Art

	Concern	Solution	Intention	Mudra for meditation	Yoga pose	Art directive
1	Ungrateful	Gratitude	"I am grateful for the support I have today."	Tarjani	Child's Pose	Begin a GRATITUDE JOURNAL, with images.
2	Distraction	Attentiveness	"I move forward with a calm body and mine."	Chinmaya	Standing Forward Bend	Draw HOW YOU ARE FEELING right now.

cont.

	Concern	Solution	Intention	Mudra for meditation	Yoga pose	Art directive
3	Instability	Stability	"Feeling my stability, I proceed with confidence."	Bhu	Mountain Pose	Paint a MOUNTAIN and a VALLEY.
4	Scattered	Concentration	"I am energized by my focused concentration".	Abhisheka	Head to Knee Forward Bend	Do a CONTOUR DRAWING, a drawing from life done without lifting the pen or pencil.
5	Unfocused	Focus	"I focus clearly as I attune to my wholeness."	Mandala	Alternate Arm and Leg Extensions	Make a MANDALA, a drawing inside a circle.

#						
6	Insecure	Security	"As I find comfort in my body, I am calm and secure."	Shankha	Cow-Cat Pose	Create a collage using COLORED TAPE.
7	Ungrounded	Groundedness	"Sitting in stillness, I am grounded."	Adhi	Goddess Pose	Do a painting on a ROCK.
8	Fearful	Fearlessness	"I am centered and I move forward in life fearlessly."	Abhaya Varada	Warrior II Pose	Make and decorate a SHIELD.

cont.

	Concern	Solution	Intention	Mudra for meditation	Yoga pose	Art directive
9	Depressed mood	Joy	"Caring for my heart, I awaken enthusiasm."	Vajrapradama	Breath of Joy	Create a STRENGTH QUILT by mounting four square-shaped drawings together, each depicting a personal strength.
10	Anxiety	Calm	"Finding peace within, I feel secure."	Pala	Legs Up The Wall Pose	Draw an INSIDE/OUTSIDE MANDALA, with images inside and outside a circle.
11	Shame	Self-acceptance	"I welcome my thoughts and feelings and embrace who I am."	Purna Hridaya	Extended Mountain Pose	Make a SELF-PORTRAIT.

			Mudra	Pose	Activity
12	Self-critical	Self-healing	"My path becomes clear as I release self-limiting beliefs."	Anamika	Puppy Pose	Do an INNER VOICE project: show what your inner voice is like with color and texture.
13	Dissociated	Embodied	"I feel at home in my body."	Prithivi	Tree Pose	Create a BODY MAP: color in a body outline using color-coding to show where different feelings are felt in the body.
14	Low self-esteem	Focus on positive qualities	"I find my inner smile and understand my inherent goodness."	Hansi	Warrior I Pose	Create a STRENGTHS COLLAGE using magazine photos showing your strengths.

cont.

	Concern	Solution	Intention	Mudra for meditation	Yoga pose	Art directive
15	Agitated	Serenity	"As I breathe, I experience serenity."	Jalashaya	Plank Pose	Make IMAGES OF FEELINGS and depict each one with paint, using color, line and texture.
16	Guilt	Innocence	"I embrace life with an open heart, and I feel acceptance."	Avahana	Sphinx Pose	Make BUBBLE PRINTS: put dish soap with watercolor in a tray. Blow bubbles with a straw and lay paper over them to create a print.

17	Anger	"I notice my inner contentment, and I live calmly."	Contentment	Chaturmukham	Half Shoulder Stand	Create an INSIDE/OUTSIDE BOX: show how you are on the inside of the box and decorate the outside showing what your outside is like.	
18	Selfishness	"I nurture my heart, and compassion blossoms."	Compassion	Padma	Camel Pose	Respond to a FAMOUS WORK OF ART.	
19	Restlessness	"I am focused and still."	Stillness	Kapota	Boat Pose	Make a CALMING LANDSCAPE, using any art material.	

cont.

	Concern	Solution	Intention	Mudra for meditation	Yoga pose	Art directive
20	Greed	Generosity	"Holding lightly, I experience ease."	Pushpanjali	Reverse Table Pose/Staff Pose	Make APPRECIATION CARDS: each person adds a visual message for the original cardholder as it is passed around the group.
21	Negativity	Positive attitude	"As I cultivate uplifting energy, I embrace life."	Prana	Side Arm Balance	Make a PICTURE OF POSITIVE THINGS in your life, using a material that you like.

| 22 | Dishonesty | Truthfulness | "Aligned with my inner self, I communicate with integrity." | Samputa | Kundalini Crow Pose | Create a BOX OF VALUES by collaging the outside with magazine images representing you. Fill the box with words cut from magazines representing what you value most. |
| 23 | Forgetful | Awareness | "I am conscious of what arises in my mind and body." | Citta | Squat Pose | Use a FOUND OBJECT as a PAINTBRUSH and make a painting. |

cont.

	Concern	Solution	Intention	Mudra for meditation	Yoga pose	Art directive
24	Stressed	Relaxation	"I release into relaxation and rest in tranquility."	Dvimukham	Corpse Pose	Create an IMAGE OF HOME: show what "home" means to you using your favorite materials.
25	Controlling	Cooperation	"I respect everyone I meet."	Anjali	Partner Chair Pose	WORK COLLABORATIVELY: find a partner and create a painting together.
26	Impulsive	Thoughtful	"Cultivating mental clarity, see my path clearly."	Jnana	Bridge Pose	Make a FUTURE SELF-PORTRAIT: what will you be like in the future? Show this in a drawing.

27	Perfectionistic	Realistic	"As I let go of control, my life becomes effortless."	Pranidhana	Lunge Pose	Make a BLINDFOLD DRAWING: yes, do a drawing while blindfolded!
28	Resistant	Openness	"I greet this day, open to possibilities."	Ushas	Seated Wide Leg Forward Bend	Create an ECCENTRIC INVENTION: solve a problem any way at all with this drawing.
29	Insensitive	Sensitivity	"As I nurture myself, I open to sensitivity."	Ida	Stork Pose	Create ART FOR OTHERS: make a piece of art to give to someone.

cont.

	Concern	Solution	Intention	Mudra for meditation	Yoga pose	Art directive
30	Uncreative	Creativity	"I connect with my creative self, and open to transformation."	Shunya	Downward Facing Dog Pose	Make a SCRIBBLE DRAWING: Make a scribble. See what it looks like and turn it into a drawing.
31	Impulsive	Careful	"As I become comfortable with myself, I cultivate care."	Svadhisthana	Forward Bend at Wall	SEW A PILLOW: Use two pieces of felt and sew the edges with embroidery floss. Stuff with fluff before sewing the final stitches.
32	Passivity	Activity	"I embrace life's vital energy."	Vittam	Dancer Pose	Make a BIG DRAWING: Tape 6 feet of butcher paper to the wall and make a picture using the whole paper!

Chapter 6

MUDRAS

The mudras suggested in the Practice Chart (Table 5.1, pages 55–66) are simply hand gestures. You may prefer to refer to them as hand gestures in situations where it is important to normalize the process with clients who are unfamiliar with yoga and meditation techniques. Typically, the word mudra refers to gestures involving the fingers and hands, but may sometimes indicate gestures of the face and body.

Mudras are common in all cultures because our dexterous hands form expressive gestures well. Think of prayer pose, peace signs, thumbs up and the OK sign, to name just a few. These gestures are part of a universal, non-verbal language. Joseph and Lillian LePage (2013) point out in their book, *Mudras for Healing and Transformation*, that mudras are tools of inner and outer communication because they allow full expression to subtle qualities for which language may be inadequate. Mudras are gestures that direct the energy in the body. According to Ramesh Shah, "mudras create inner peace and inner strength, eliminate fatigue and anxiety, protect physical and emotional health, help transcend stress, depression, guilt and anger, calm the mind and sharpen intuition" (Menen 2010, p.11). The qualities brought out by the mudras are inherent in every person; performing a mudra in conjunction with an intention allows you to choose consciously to feel and express that quality. Mudras are an aid to translating intentions into action and as such can be a bridge between inner experience and outer interactions.

Hand mudras are powerful because of the sensory and motor nerve endings present in the fingers and hands. The gestures provide a range of possibilities for how the energy is channeled to the brain and the rest of the body. The LePages refer to each mudra as having "core qualities" (2013, p.8) or inherent positive qualities that relate to qualities already present in our nature as humans. They identify mudras as tools for health and healing because with conscious use mudras support the awakening and integration of our inherent positive qualities. Physically, mudras direct awareness and allow a person to perceive breath and physical sensation more readily. Mudras are also understood to direct what yogis call "prana" or life force energy, along energy pathways in the subtle body. These effects can be felt on a psychological level, supporting a range of psycho-emotional qualities ranging from calming to energizing and affecting confidence, self-esteem and vitality, among many other feelings.

Mudras are an ideal practice for linking with art therapy. Both art making and practicing mudras are forms of self-expression. In mudra making, the hands take on sculptural shapes that hold metaphoric meaning, a natural connection to art therapy. A skilled art therapist chooses art materials and interventions in a similar manner as one might choose an appropriate mudra – in response to the client's needs, often in the interest of creating balance and integration. Both mudras and art are forms of non-verbal communication. In art therapy the art is seen as a reflection of what is already present for the client/artist. Likewise, mudras amplify qualities already present in a person. Much as an art therapist expects the act of creating art to address issues in a way that words cannot, consciously creating the shape of a mudra translates intention into a physical form (McGonigal 2008). Mudras are easy to learn and can be done in almost any setting and any population. Even people who are very reluctant to move their bodies into yoga poses will usually be willing to try a hand gesture.

Mudra instructions and qualities

The mudras' numbers correspond to the rows on the chart. Mudras can be performed while standing, sitting (in a chair or on the floor), or even lying down. The person practicing the mudra should simply be relaxed and alert. When guiding someone in the use of mudras, begin by asking the person to use full breaths. After describing the gesture, ask the person to find a long spine and relax their shoulders.

1. Tarjani

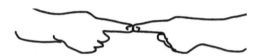

With palms facing the torso, extend both index fingers and allow the tips to touch, folding all the other fingers in. (Modification for long fingernails: interlock index fingers and tug gently.)

QUALITIES: Supports heart opening, cultivating self-acceptance, gratitude, compassion and harmony.

2. Chinmaya

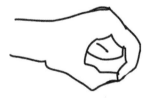

With palms facing downward connect the first finger and thumb of each hand, forming a circle and then fold all other fingers inward. Rest the whole shape on thighs.

QUALITIES: Grounding, balance, sense of support, serenity, security.

3. Bhu

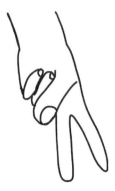

Extend middle and index fingers of both hands out to a "V" shape. Curl ring and little fingers inward and place thumbs on top. Seated on the floor, extend arms to the sides and press the tips of the index and middle fingers on the floor.

QUALITIES: Stability, embodiment, security, emotional stability, trust.

4. Abhisheka

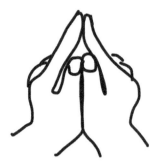

With palms facing one another make loose fists and join the heels of the hands and knuckles then extend the index fingers and let their tips meet, while allowing the inner edges of the thumbs to meet. The thumbs then rest in the space between the fingers.

QUALITIES: Concentration, clarity, focus, meditation.

5. Mandala

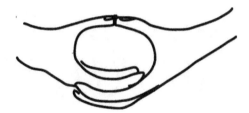

With palms facing upwards, and fingers pointing inward, rest the right hand on top of the left. Allow the tips of the thumbs to meet, forming a circular shape.

QUALITIES: Unity, completeness, wholeness, integration.

6. Shankha

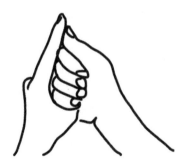

With palms facing up rest the right hand on top of the left. Then allow the four fingers of the right hand to grasp the left thumb. Touch the tip of the left index finger to the tip of the right thumb. Rest the whole shape on the lap.

QUALITIES: Safety, contentment, stress reduction, inner nourishment.

7. Adhi

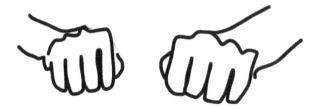

With palms facing down, form loose fists around the thumbs of both hands. Rest the shapes on the thighs.

QUALITIES: Stillness, support, structure, tranquility.

8. Abhaya Varada

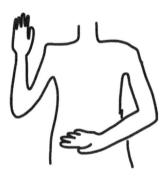

With palm facing up, rest the left hand in the lap or cup it just below the navel. With palm facing away from the torso bring the right hand to shoulder level, slightly cupped. Right fingertips point upward while the right elbow rests comfortably near the waist.

QUALITIES: Fearlessness, centering, anxiety reduction, presence.

9. Vajrapradama

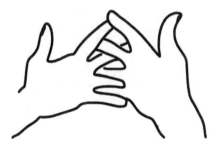

Loosely interlace the fingers with the palms facing upwards and the left little finger on the bottom. Extend the thumbs and angle all the fingers slightly upward while holding the shape a hand's width away from the torso at chest level. Hold elbows slightly away from the body.

QUALITIES: Confidence, enthusiasm, self-trust, vitality.

10. Pala

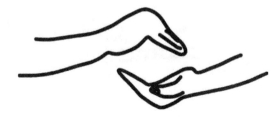

Cup the left hand and place it palm up below the navel with the little finger lightly touching the low abdomen. Cup the right hand and place it palm down above the left hand with thumb lightly touching the abdomen at navel level.

QUALITIES: Anti-anxiety, calm, trust, tranquility.

11. Purna Hridaya

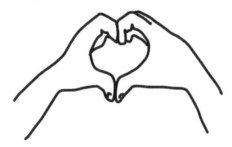

With hands facing downwards, interlace the fingertips with the right index finger closest to the chest. Curl the fingers as you bring the thumb prints together, thumbs stretching downward. The hands form the shape of the heart and the shape is held in front of the sternum.

QUALITIES: Acceptance, emotional awareness, heart opening, love.

12. Anamika

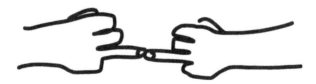

With palms facing the abdomen, gently connect the tips of the ring fingers and fold all other fingers inward. Alternatively, interlock ring fingers and tug gently.

QUALITIES: Healing, self-assurance, comfort, support of healthy relationships.

13. Prithivi

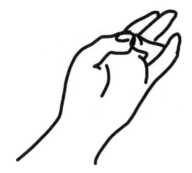

With palms facing up, connect the tips of the ring fingers and thumbs. Extend all other fingers and rest the backs of the hands on the thighs.

QUALITIES: Security, grounding, embodiment, confidence.

14. Hansi

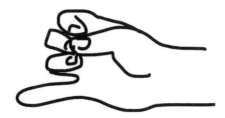

With palms facing up bring the tips of the thumbs together with the tips of the first three fingers on each hand. Extend the little fingers and place the shape on the thighs.

QUALITIES: Bliss, joy, lightness, optimism.

15. Jalashaya

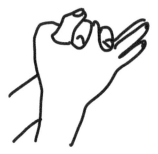

Interlace the fingers with the right thumb on top. Extend the ring and little fingers so they point away from the body while the heels of the hands rest below the navel.

QUALITIES: Calming, cooling, soothing, balancing.

16. Avahana

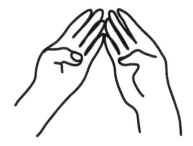

With palms facing up and the fingers together, touch the tip of each thumb to the base of the ring finger. Keep the palms flat and allow the outer tips of the ring and little fingers to touch. With arms bent at the elbow, let the forearms touch the abdomen.

QUALITIES: Acceptance, optimism, compassion, learning.

17. Chaturmukham

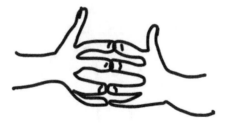

With palms facing and fingers rounded, allow the tips of all the fingers to meet the fingertips on the opposite hand. Fingers are separated and the thumbs point upwards. Lightly rest the wrists on the abdomen.

QUALITIES: Contentment, positive attitude, completeness, sense of ease.

18. Padma

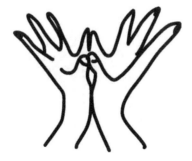

With palms facing, place the base of the palms together and open the fingers wide. Allow the inside of the thumbs and the outside edge of the little fingers to touch. Hold this shape in front of the chest, fingers pointing upwards.

QUALITIES: Cultivates unconditional love, empathy, balanced awareness, patience.

19. Kapota

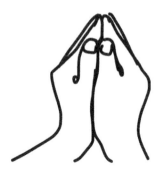

With palms facing, press the heels of the hands together, let the fingertips touch and seal the inner edges of the thumbs. Keeping this, bend the fingers to create a hollow area between the palms. Hold the shape at the center of the chest.

QUALITIES: Peacefulness, introspection, unity, obedience.

20. Pushpanjali

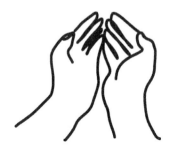

With palms facing up, cup the hands keeping the fingers together and allow the outer tips of the ring and little finger to touch. Elbows rest against the abdomen and the hands move away from the body, as if making an offering.

QUALITIES: Offering, releasing attachments, appreciation, generosity.

21. Prana

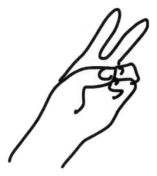

With palms facing up extend the index fingers and middle fingers in a "v" shape while connecting the tips of the thumbs with the ring and little fingers. Rest the backs of the hands on the thighs.

QUALITIES: Energizing, joy, vibrancy, vitality.

22. Samputa

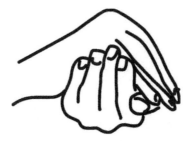

With palm facing up, cup the left hand and hold it at navel level. With palm facing down, cup the right hand and place it over the left; the heel of the hand rests on the left little finger edge of the hand and the fingertips rest on the edge of the left thumb, creating a hollow area between the hands.

QUALITIES: Integrity, truthfulness, safety, valuing the self.

23. Citta

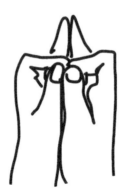

With palms facing one another, extend the middle, ring and little fingers. Connect the thumb tips to the tips of the index fingers and bring the hands together so that the edges of the thumbs come together and the tips of the index fingers touch each other. The other fingers point upwards and the shape is held at chest level with elbows slightly away from the body.

QUALITIES: Supports concentration, discernment, mental clarity, objectivity.

24. Dvimukham

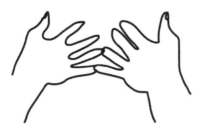

With palms facing upwards, allow the tips of the little fingers and ring fingers to touch those of the opposite hand. Fingers are held loosely apart from one another and the shape rests on the lap with the forearms resting against the abdomen.

QUALITIES: Supports relaxation, stress reduction, tranquility.

25. Anjali

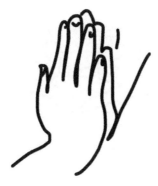

Palms and fingers meet with thumbs facing the chest and fingers pointing up. Hold the shape in front of the chest with elbows slightly away from the sides of the abdomen.

QUALITIES: Devotion, reverence, unity, inner silence, calms the mind, known as the gesture of offering.

26. Jnana

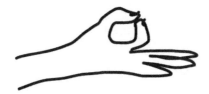

With palms facing upward, allow the index finger and thumb tips to meet on each hand, forming a circle. Extend the other fingers and rest the shape on the thighs.

QUALITIES: Clarity, wisdom, intuitive knowledge, limitlessness.

27. Pranidhana

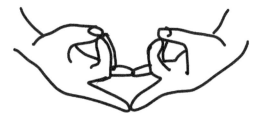

With palms facing upwards bring the thumbs to touch the middle and ring fingers of each hand. Then extend the index and little fingers and allow the tips to meet those of the opposite hand. Allow the backs of the wrist to rest in the lap with thumbs, middle and ring fingertips pointing up.

QUALITIES: Surrender, release, relaxation, releasing attachments.

28. Ushas

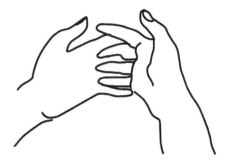

With palms facing up, the fingers loosely interlace and the shape rests on the lap.

QUALITIES: Open to possibility, harmony, curiosity, positive attitude.

29. Ida

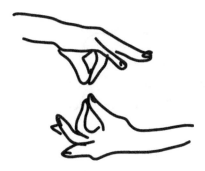

With palm facing upward bring the ring finger and thumb of the left hand to meet and extend the other fingers. Place that shape near the abdomen, just below the navel. Bring the right palm to face downwards and join the thumb and ring fingers and extend the other fingers. Arrange the right hand so that the joined fingers of the right hand are directly above those of the left hand without touching.

QUALITIES: Receptivity, awareness, fluidity, pleasure, sensitivity, balance.

30. Shunya

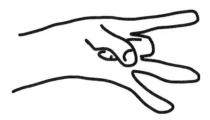

With palms facing up, fold the middle fingers in toward the base of the thumb and use the thumbs to gently hold them down. Extend the other fingers and place the backs of the hands on the thighs.

QUALITIES: Openness, tension release, awakening intuition, attunement.

31. Svadhisthana

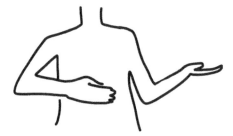

With palm facing up, cup the left hand and bring it to navel level, away from the body and angled to the side, with elbow at the side of the abdomen and forearm parallel to the ground. The right hand is cupped and placed below the navel with the palm facing the low abdomen.

QUALITIES: Wholeness, self-nourishment, fluidity, sensuality, security.

32. Vittam

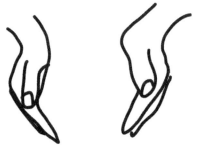

With palms facing bring the hands at the level of the low abdomen, slightly cupped. Hands are about a foot apart, the distance varies with the natural movement of inhalation (hands move apart) and exhalation (hands move together).

QUALITIES: Vitality, energizing, healing.

Chapter 7

MEDITATION

Mindfulness meditation

There are many forms of meditation. Sometimes people are reluctant to try meditation because of a misconception that a meditator must be able to clear the mind of thoughts. This may be a goal of some forms of advanced meditation practice, but in general the purpose of meditation is to practice witnessing thoughts, feelings, sensations, really all aspects of being, without judgment. The accessible form of meditation that is suggested in this book is based on what is known as mindfulness meditation.

Mindfulness meditation simply means that one engages and quiets the mind by becoming "mindful" (Rappaport and Kalmanowitz 2014, p.24). To be mindful a person uses awareness to notice any aspect of the self that the mind might go to with an attitude of acceptance. Using awareness with acceptance means that the meditator trains the self to avoid getting involved with the opinions the mind generates. Instead, the meditator uses non-judgmental observation. Where a person is on the continuum of ability is not important. The benefit comes from practicing. Every time we practice releasing judgment in meditation we have a model for how we can do so in life. Every time we release judgment of ourselves and others we are able to see behavior more clearly and therefore are more able to make conscious choices. In mindfulness meditation the attention can rest on any object. Examples might be the breath, a candle flame, sounds or a mantra. In yoga and art mudra meditation the intention becomes a mantra, or a word or phrase that repeats. Thoughts will come and go. As one becomes the observer, cultivating that position with practice, gradually one learns to witness it all: thoughts, feelings, sensations from the calm still position of the inner observer, accepting and not judging.

Jon Kabat-Zinn (2005), the well-known meditation teacher, says in *Wherever You Go, There You Are*:

> To let go means to give up coercing, resisting, or struggling, in exchange for something more powerful and wholesome which comes out of allowing things to be as they are without getting caught up in your attraction to or rejection of them, in the intrinsic stickiness of wanting, of liking and disliking. (p.53)

He describes mindfulness as staying in the present moment on purpose, non-judgmentally.

Meditation does not mean that you will have to stop your thoughts. It is likely that some activities you already do give access to the meditator's witness position. Whenever we experience an act without involving self-criticism and self-consciousness we are accessing that sweet inner observer. Some find that sports, art making, practicing crafts, engaging in play or even singing in the shower might give them moments of mindfulness. To cultivate the ability to behave mindfully means we gain access to our emotional and physical sensations while witnessing our experience with compassion. To behave as a witness in place of being critical, gives us a powerful tool to transform how we choose to react to experiences.

Meditation links well to art therapy because making art in an art therapy context carries the same mindful sense of observing and making conscious choices by learning from your observations (Rappaport and Kalmanowitz 2014). The more one can make art mindfully, without self-conscious judgment, the better able the artist is to find the flow state that generates the benefits associated with art therapy such as self-soothing, increased endorphins or enhanced self-esteem. Shaun McNiff speaks of using art mindfully to access all aspects of our psyches, looking at art using what he calls "witness consciousness," and deepening conventional mindfulness practices (McNiff 2014, p.38). Pat Allen aptly connects intention and witness to the act of making art. Artists who learn to meditate deepen their understanding of mindfulness. Meditation develops the tools of intention and witnessing. When these tools are applied to art making they enhance the art's ability to bridge the unconscious with the conscious (Allen 2014).

How to create a meditation

To create and practice a meditation using the Practice Chart for Intention Centered Yoga and Art (Table 5.1) begin with the intention. The intention should be customized so that the person using it finds it both resonant and easy to remember, as discussed in Chapter 3. Next, find a comfortable seat. This can be sitting on the floor or on a chair. If seated on the floor it is helpful to have the hips elevated by sitting on the edge of a folded blanket, several blankets or a yoga block. The aim is to allow the knees to rest comfortably on the floor and the spine to find its natural curves and length. Some people may find it comfortable to bring their back against a wall. A chair works well also, adjusted so that the feet can be flat on the floor and the shoulders remain over the hips, again to form the natural curves of the spine and find length without discomfort. It might be useful to place a pillow between the natural curve of the lumbar spine and the back of the chair. Aligned posture allows the body to support itself without excess muscular energy and allows for greater relaxation and comfort. Keeping the spine lifted, as if there were a string at the top of the head, assisting in the lift, relax the shoulders. Assume the selected mudra. Allow the eyes to close, or relax the gaze by angling the eyes downward to find a spot on which to rest the gaze. Next, allow the breath to deepen and scan the body for any residual tension. Breathe consciously and allow tension to release on the exhale. At this point an optional practice is to say to yourself or aloud to those you are guiding, "relax your body," "relax your mind," "relax your emotions." Take a slow breath between each phrase and savor these moments as a chance to leave behind anything that is not needed. Take a moment to notice what effects the mudra has for you, your body and breath. When a comfortable rhythm of full breathing is established, repeat the intention aloud three times. Continue to hold the mudra and allow the intention to repeat silently in the mind, following the rhythm of the breath. The cadence of the words is established by the meditator, perhaps repeated once on the inhale and again on the exhale, or some may prefer to break the chosen phrase into two parts, matching half the phrase to the inhale, and half to the exhale. Continue with the established pattern for one to ten minutes.

People who are new to meditation should begin with short durations and lengthen the time as is comfortable. Experienced meditators may wish to follow this pattern for up to 30 minutes. Alternatively, once the mantra/intention has been established, some may wish to shift the object of meditation (after about five minutes) to inner silence, by either following the breath or by observing the qualities of the mudra and how its effects are felt in the body. Remember to remain a simple witness by avoiding any judgment. Of course, for all meditators, thoughts come in, the mind may wander or judgments intrude. This is to be expected! Consider each occurrence another opportunity to practice compassionate consciousness; gently notice what is happening and return to the object of your mindful observation without self-admonishment, but instead with friendly encouragement.

Design the meditation for success. Brief meditations have many benefits: a person will not be intimidated by the prospect of sitting still for long periods, and it fits into busy schedules. Experiencing the success of a short meditation may then lead naturally to extending the time in subsequent sessions. Keep the individual or group's needs and capabilities in mind. When guiding a group to meditate, do practice along with the group but do not close your eyes. It is your job to observe the reactions of the group members so that you can guide or adjust accordingly. Groups generally benefit from shorter meditations, at times simply using the practice of the mudra and repeating the intention aloud as a means of establishing the focus of the group. In the case of shorter meditations the duration can be measured by counting breaths rather than in minutes.

For example, you may decide that your group would benefit from an improved ability to focus. The group begins by establishing the theme of "focus." You suggest an intention and possibly use the group's input to find the best wording that feels natural and true for the group members. Something like, "I can focus clearly, as I calm my breath." Next you would show the participants how to assume Mandala mudra. When everyone has their hands arranged, then have them sit tall with feet flat on the floor, relax their shoulders and deepen the breath. Then say "Repeat after me…" and recite the intention. Repeat this process two more times or have them join you in two more repetitions. After that you ask them to repeat the intention silently to themselves. Request that the group members continue to repeat silently the intention for a number of slow breaths, likely one to ten breaths, (ten average breaths equals about one minute). You then complete the meditation by guiding the group to take a final deep breath, inhaling through the nose and exhaling through the mouth (a "deep cleansing breath").

For a longer meditation begin in the same manner, repeating the intention, and then ask the meditators to shift to observing the effects of the mudra while simultaneously noticing the breath entering and leaving the body. It may be helpful to suggest a point of observation such as the nostrils, noticing the sensation of the breath entering and leaving the nostrils. Alternatively, one can observe the breath at the belly, in the lungs, or by noticing the rising and falling of the chest.

BRIEF INTENTION CENTERED MEDITATION

1. Sit tall with spine erect and feet flat on the floor (or in a comfortable cross-legged position).

2. Assume the selected mudra and relax the shoulders with an exhale.

3. Take a deep cleansing breath – inhale deeply through the nose, exhale through the mouth then establish slow steady breathing.

4. Repeat the chosen intention aloud three times.

5. Break the chosen intention into two parts (example: "I am"/ "whole and beautiful."). Repeat the intention, silently, with the breath (example: inhale "I am," exhale "whole and beautiful.").

6. Continue for ten breaths.

7. End with a deep cleansing breath.

Chapter 8

YOGA POSES

Much as mudras have energetic effects on the body and mind, so too do yoga postures. For the purposes of this book I have selected basic yoga poses that one can find descriptions and instructions for in many readily available sources. Yoga teachers of different traditions may have different names for them. In Sanskrit, the language generally used in yogic tradition, the poses are called asana. I will use the term poses in an effort to keep all aspects of the practice accessible. Yoga has become popular and widely practiced in the Western world. While it is wonderful that this transformative practice is readily available to everyone, a word of caution is in order. If you are a clinician please remember to stay within your scope of practice and recognize when further training is required. Please use trusted sources of information and begin with the simplest version of a pose for yourself and your clients. Remember that you are practicing yoga or incorporating poses into your clinical practice because of the benefits yoga can offer. The benefits are not available if pain or stress are induced.

Finding your edge

In any yoga practice it is advisable to avoid pain, but that does not mean to avoid sensation. Discriminate between the sensation of muscles stretching or working, and pain. Attention to the breath is the perfect guide. If a person must hold their breath, is panting or unable to breathe smoothly then it is time to ease off the depth of the pose. At the same time it is important to be fully engaged. Think of giving every pose 80 percent effort. Engagement of 80 percent is your edge. If you are so engaged, you can continue practicing without exhaustion. Effort of 100 percent cannot be maintained. Fifty percent effort allows the mind to wander and may cause the person to be careless about physical alignment.

While practicing, there is a natural tendency to compare your pose to that of another person. It is tempting to try to force your body into a different expression of the pose than it might be capable of at the time. We all have images of yogis using their bodies to create shapes like pretzels. Strength, flexibility, body type, fitness level, duration of practice and personal history all contribute to the body's ability to assume poses. In general, those who are quite flexible need to gain strength in order to find balance and alignment. Those who are very muscular are more balanced when they gain flexibility. The purpose of yoga practice is not to achieve any particular level of fitness, flexibility or strength. While these may be wonderful side effects of a dedicated practice the real reason to practice yoga is for the benefits. The benefits of practicing yoga are a clear, calm mind and enhanced self-awareness. These qualities are what some call the "yoga high" which can happen for everyone when they come to the practice with sincere engagement. The yogis who assume seemingly impossible shapes do so to work their edge, the place where they can maintain full engagement, in order to receive the benefits. You receive the very same benefits by practicing at your own edge. Pattabhi Jois, the founder of Ashtanga yoga famously said, "Practice and all is coming" (Awaken 2013).

Matching breath to movement and keeping the body properly aligned may be achieved and maintained with full engagement. Bringing attention to the practice without competition or judgment generates mindfulness. A mindful practice is most likely to have a broad impact beyond the yoga and art session.

Directions for all poses

Establish steady deep breathing before you begin. Use the breath as you move into the pose as well as when you maintain the pose. In other words, always move with a breath. A yoga instructor will have preferences for which movements occur on the inhale and which on the exhale. For the purposes of this book it is more important for you to find the breath that feels natural to you and to breathe purposefully. Generally it is a good idea to begin to establish the breath in Mountain Pose (page 96) and move from there. If the pose is on the floor begin in a simple Tabletop Pose (page 94) with knees under the hips and hands shoulder width, directly under the shoulders and spine long and level.

Contraindications: There may be contraindications for some poses such as high blood pressure, glaucoma, head or eye injuries or other health concerns. Please consult a medical professional if any of these conditions are present and follow their advice. In general, if there is doubt use an alternative pose that does not bring the head below the heart. Ideally, you will have a yoga teacher or trusted resource from which to gain more information about each pose. Finding alignment and feeling the pose in many parts of the body is important as the practitioner gains experience and sensitivity. The instructions given here are simple and basic. Please do not share a pose with a client or anyone else unless you have experienced it in your own body. If you have questions or doubts of any kind then seek out a registered yoga instructor who can give specific advice. There are many online sources for yoga information. *Yoga Journal* (2014) online is extensive and reliable in the quality of information, as are others. Remember that every person's body is different and has different history and sensitivities. There is no single correct way to do a pose.

In Intention Centered Yoga and Art Practice no specialized equipment is needed. A yoga mat, a block and a strap might be nice, but are not necessary in order to perform any of the poses listed here. For modifications it is helpful to have a folded blanket and an armless chair.

Yoga pose instructions and qualities

1a. Tabletop Pose

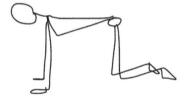

1. Child's Pose

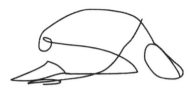

Begin in **Tabletop Pose** on hands and knees with knees directly under the hips and wrists directly under the shoulders and then sit back on the heels. Bring the forehead to the floor and the hands to the sides. If head does not reach the floor or the seat does not reach the heels then prop with a folded blanket. If full flexion bothers the knees then place a blanket snug behind both knees.

ALTERNATIVE: Seated Chair Forward Bend
Sit in a chair with feet flat on the floor, hip width apart, and fold the torso over the thighs. Arms can drape toward the floor or be folded to support the head. The chair could also be at a table and folded arms support the forehead. A deeper expression of the pose would be **Seated Forward Bend**: Begin seated on the floor with legs extended parallel to one another and feet flexed. Reach arms overhead and extend the spine. Tip forward from the hips, keeping spine straight and reach hands toward the toes. Relax the head toward the legs. If the lower back rounds please use a folded blanket under the seat.

QUALITIES: Calming, grounding, inward focusing, restful, stress relieving, humbling.

2. Standing Forward Bend

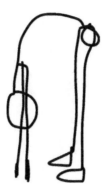

Begin in **Mountain Pose** (see 3, on page 96), with feet hipbone distance apart, bend the knees slightly and roll the torso over the legs. Bring the head down so that the crown of the head faces the floor. Place hands on the floor, on blocks or clasp opposite elbows.

ALTERNATIVE: Seated Chair Forward Bend
Sit in a chair with feet flat on the floor, hip width apart, and fold the torso over the thighs. Arms can drape toward the floor or be folded to support the head. The chair could also be at a table and folded arms support the forehead. A deeper expression of the pose would be **Seated Forward Bend**: Begin seated on the floor with legs extended parallel to one another and feet flexed. Reach arms overhead and extend the spine. Tip forward from the hips, keeping spine straight and reach hands toward the toes. Relax the head toward the legs. If the lower back rounds please use a folded blanket under the seat.

QUALITIES: Calms the brain, reduces fatigue, reduces anxiety, stress relieving, focusing.

3. Mountain Pose

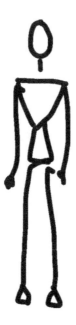

Stand with feet hip width apart, second toes parallel to one another. Find your weight evenly balanced on the feet. While rooting down with the feet lift up through the crown of the head. Firm the thighs and lift the knee caps, lift the sternum, bring the chin parallel to the floor. Relax the shoulders, let the arms be energetic at your sides. Lengthen the tailbone toward the floor. Align the ears over the shoulders, the shoulders over the hips and the hips over the ankles.

ALTERNATIVE: Seated Mountain Pose
Sit on a chair with feet flat on the floor, hip width apart. Find the seat square on the sit bones and lift through the crown of the head. Lift the navel, lift the sternum, relax the shoulders. Bring the chin level to the ground and square the ears over the shoulders and the shoulders over the hips. Hands rest face down on the thighs if seated in a chair or palms are placed on the floor on either side of hips.

QUALITIES: Improves self-esteem, enhances confidence, grounding, stability, strength.

4. Head to Knee Forward Bend

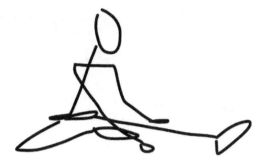

Sit on the floor with a folded blanket lifting your buttocks, legs stretched out with the toes pointing up. Fold the right leg in so the sole of the foot rests on the inner upper thigh of the opposite leg. The knee of the outstretched leg can bend slightly or be supported with a folded blanket. Press the hands on the floor on either side of the left leg and turn the torso slightly to the left. Reach the spine long and tip forward from the pelvis and begin to lay the belly on the thigh, coming down slowly and only as far as is comfortable. Repeat on the opposite side.

ALTERNATIVE: Forward Bend at Wall (see 31, page 124)
Begin facing the wall in **Mountain Pose** (see 3, page 96), 12 inches away from the wall. Place your palms against the wall a little above waist height, shoulder width apart. Walk the feet back as you press your hands to the wall until the body forms an "L" shape. The arms and torso form a straight line with the head between the upper arms, crown of the head facing the wall. Engage the legs with knees slightly bent, quadriceps lifting. Lift the navel as you lengthen the torso and engage the arms. Move shoulders away from the ears as you broaden across the chest.

QUALITIES: Focus, equanimity, balance, concentration.

5. Alternate Arm and Leg Extensions

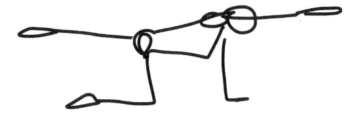

Begin in **Tabletop Pose**, on hands and knees with knees directly under the hips and wrists directly under the shoulders. Extend the right arm and left leg parallel to the ground. Keep toes pointing down and thumb pointing up with fingers extended. Lift and engage the navel while lengthening from crown to tail. The gaze rests on the floor between the hands. Place arm and leg back to starting position and extend the opposite arm and leg in the same manner. Repeat, moving with the breath.

ALTERNATIVE: Standing Alternate Arm and Leg Extensions
Begin facing the wall, arms length away, with palms flat on wall at shoulder height, feet hip width with second toes parallel to one another. Lift and extend the right arm overhead while simultaneously lifting the right knee. As the arm extends, pay attention to the opposite foot grounding and providing stability. Extend the torso, and lift and engage the navel. Return to start position and repeat the movement with the opposite arm and leg.

ALTERNATIVE: Seated Alternate Arm and Leg Extensions
This pose could also be done seated, alternately lifting arms straight overhead while focusing on the opposite sit bone and sole of foot grounding and providing stability.

QUALITIES: Focus, centering, balance, locating internal compass.

6. Cow-Cat Pose

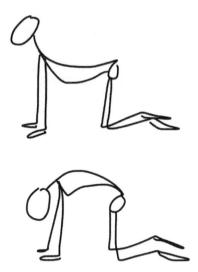

Begin on hands and knees in **Tabletop Pose** with a neutral spine; hips directly over knees and shoulders directly over the wrists. Spread the fingers and press down with the whole hand. Toes are pointed directly behind the knees and tops of the feet press down. Leading with the tailbone, begin to flex the spine first by dropping the belly and rolling shoulders onto the back and lifting the chin. Then tip the tail downwards, lift the navel toward the spine, round the shoulders and bring the chin toward the chest. Repeat, following the breath.

ALTERNATIVE: Seated Spinal Flexion
Sit on a chair with feet flat on the floor, hip distance apart, parallel to one another. Bring hands to the thighs or knees with arms straight, spine long, sitting tall. Inhale and lift the chin and the chest, rolling shoulders back. Exhale and round the shoulders, bring chin to chest and pull navel toward the spine. Use the strength of the arms to facilitate the movement in this pose.

QUALITIES: Heart opening, balancing, enhances flexibility, enhances open-mindedness, stability, security.

7. Goddess Pose

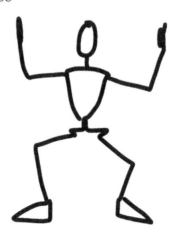

With hands on hips step the feet about four feet apart. Turn toes out at 45-degree angles, and then bend knees carefully tracking the knees over the ankles. Engage the core by making the spine erect with the navel lifted and the tailbone moving toward the floor. Crown of the head lifts toward the ceiling and gaze is straight ahead. Bring the arms out to the sides at shoulder level. Turn palms up and relax shoulders away from the ears. Finally, bend arms at the elbow so that fingers point toward the ceiling and then spread fingers wide and turn palms to face forward.

ALTERNATIVE: Seated Goddess Pose

Seated in a chair with feet flat on the floor, come to the edge of the seat and bring feet three to four feet apart at 45-degree angles. Press feet firmly to the ground as you engage the core by making the spine erect with the navel lifted and the tailbone moving toward the floor. Crown of the head lifts toward the ceiling and gaze is straight ahead. Bring the arms out to the sides at shoulder level. Turn palms up and relax shoulders away from the ears. Finally, bend arms at the elbow so that fingers point toward the ceiling and then spread fingers wide and turn palms to face forward.

QUALITIES: Confidence, stability, strength, poise, groundedness.

8. Warrior II Pose

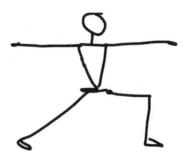

Begin by stepping the feet about four feet apart. Bring the hands to the hips and turn the right foot out to the right and turn the left foot to 90 degrees. The heel of the right foot should line up with the instep of the left. Carefully bend the right knee, tracking the knee over the ankle. Do not over bend the knee; it should not go past the heel. If the knee needs to bend deeper, make the space between the feet longer. Allow the hips to open and keep the left leg strong and straight. Square the shoulders over the hips and extend the arms at shoulder level, palms facing down with fingers together. Lift and engage through the core by lifting the navel in and up, while allowing the tailbone to descend toward the floor. Relax the shoulders, engage the arms and turn the gaze to look over the right fingertips. Repeat on the opposite side.

ALTERNATIVE: Chair Warrior II Pose
Come in to the pose as above, but with an armless chair waiting, seat facing the right thigh. As you come to bend the right leg, position the chair to support the thigh and right sit bone. Allow the hips to open and keep the left leg strong and straight. Square the shoulders over the hips and extend the arms at shoulder level, palms facing down with fingers together. Lift and engage through the core by lifting the navel in and up, while allowing the tailbone to descend toward the floor. Relax the shoulders, engage the arms and turn the gaze to look over the right fingertips. Repeat on the opposite side.

QUALITIES: Courage, strength, open to new experiences, stamina, perseverance.

9. Breath of Joy

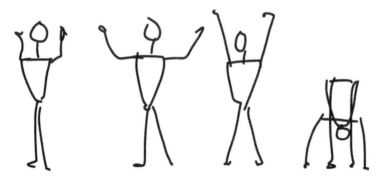

This is the name for a flow that combines breath and movement that can be done in a variety of ways. One way is to stand with feet hip width apart, parallel to one another. Take a three-part inhale by sniffing in through the nose and retaining the breath between sniffs. Arms take a different position with each sniff, first extended out at shoulder level about 45 degrees to the body, next bring the arms slightly closer and higher, now fingers pointing to where the wall and the ceiling meet. Each sniff is a sip of air approximately equal to one third lung capacity. On the last sniff complete the inhale and bring arms enthusiastically above the head, fingers pointing toward the ceiling. Exhale powerfully with the sound of "ha!" as you sweep the arms toward the floor, bending at the waist and bending slightly at the knees. Repeat right away, sweeping the arms to the first position with a sniff. Repeat the entire sequence five to nine times.

ALTERNATIVE: Seated Breath of Joy
Repeat the arm positions and breathe while seated in a chair with feet flat on the floor. Instead of forward folding on the exhale, allow the arms to drop into the lap, palms up.

QUALITIES: Stress relieving, uplifts mood, enhances joy, energizing.

10. Legs Up The Wall Pose

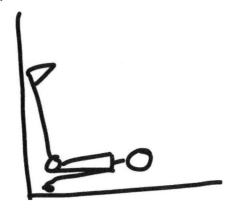

Begin by sitting next to the wall with the right hip touching the wall. Keeping as close to the wall as possible, lean back and swing the legs up the wall. You will end up lying on your back with the torso perpendicular to the wall and the legs together and extended toward the ceiling. You may be able to scoot toward the wall until the sit bones touch it, but it is fine to have the buttocks a few inches from the wall. If desired a folded blanket or bolster may be placed under the sacrum and low back, generally higher if you are more flexible, less high if you are stiffer.

ALTERNATIVE: Modified Corpse Pose
Lie on the floor and bring the lower legs onto the seat of a chair. Legs should be 90 degrees at the hips and the knees. If adjustment is needed for height, put blankets under the torso, or if knees seem too high then place a folded blanket on the seat of the chair. As an option you may use a yoga strap around the thighs to keep the knees in line with the hips without effort. Roll shoulders comfortably onto the back and relax the body.

QUALITIES: Calms the mind, relieves anxiety and depressive symptoms, soothing, grounding.

11. Extended Mountain Pose

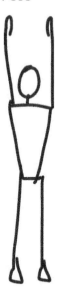

Begin in **Mountain Pose** (see 3, page 96), and then raise the arms overhead, perpendicular to the floor with palms facing and fingers stretching up. Straighten arms and lower shoulders away from the ears.

ALTERNATIVE: If shoulders are tight, then only raise arms as far as it is comfortable, focusing on keeping arms parallel to one another without hunching shoulders. The pose may be done seated in a chair as well.

QUALITIES: Relieves anxiety, energizing, promotes determination, acceptance.

12. Puppy Pose

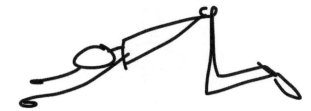

Begin on hands and knees in **Tabletop Pose**, with hands under shoulders and knees directly under the hips, tops of feet on the floor, directly behind the knees. Walk the hands away from you on the floor as you drop the chest and forehead to the floor. You may want to put one or more folded blankets under the forehead and chest for comfort. Keep the hips over the knees.

ALTERNATIVE: Modified Downward Dog Pose
Stand in **Mountain Pose** (see 3, page 96) in front of a table. Keep lower body strongly in place as you walk hands forward on the table. Gently fold at the hips as you lower chest and forehead to the table. A blanket may be used here as well.

QUALITIES: Calms the mind, stress relieving, energizing, enhances flexibility.

13. Tree Pose

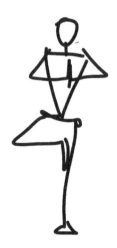

Begin in **Mountain Pose** (see 3, page 96). Shift the weight to the right foot and bend the left knee and then bring the sole of the foot to one of three positions. Draw the sole of the left foot to press the right inner thigh, inner shin or place the toes on the floor and bring the sole of the foot to the inner right ankle. Place hands on the hips, in Anjali mudra (see 25, page 81), or reach the arms overhead. Repeat on the opposite side.

ALTERNATIVE: One of the choices above will be appropriate for most people. The pose may be done with the back to a wall where the buttocks and shoulders lightly touch for secure balance.

QUALITIES: Balance, concentration, embodiment, stability, supports confidence.

14. Warrior I Pose

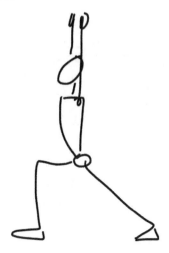

Begin in **Mountain Pose** (see 3, page 96), with hands on hips, step the left leg back about three and a half feet, keeping the feet hip width apart. Turn the left foot outward 45 degrees and bend the right knee, tracking the knee directly over the ankle. Keep the shoulders over the hips and keep the hips facing forward. If it feels right, raise the arms overhead with fingers extended and palms facing. Relax the shoulders away from the ears. Repeat on the second side.

ALTERNATIVE: As you step into the pose, place an armless chair under the thigh and sit bone for support.

QUALITIES: Focus, balance, stability, improves self-esteem.

15. Plank Pose

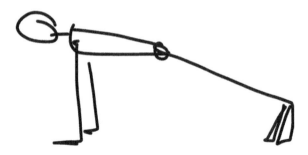

Come to hands and knees in **Tabletop Pose**. Stretch the right leg back with toes curled under and heel pressing back. Holding that, stretch the left leg back as well, creating a straight line from the crown of the head to the heels. Engage the navel and keep arms straight without locking the elbows.

ALTERNATIVE: Assume the pose with both knees on the floor, keeping the straight line between the crown of the head and the knees. Or, place a block at the pubic bone to support the body, while maintaining alignment.

QUALITIES: Inner strength, stabilization, serenity, willpower.

16. Sphinx Pose

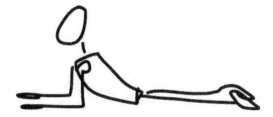

Lie down on the stomach. Lift the chest as you draw bent elbows under the shoulders and extend the forearms parallel to one another, palms down and fingers extended. Press the tops of the feet down, hip width apart. The shoulders roll back as the navel lifts, engaging the core, and isometrically tug the hands back toward the body. The chin is parallel to the ground and the shoulders relax away from the ears. Press the pubic bone at the front of the pelvis to the floor and lift the navel to avoid lower back pressure.

ALTERNATIVE: Seated Sphinx Pose
Seated in a chair at a table, bring the forearms to the table, shoulder width apart, palms down, fingers spread. Proceed as above, but instead of pressing the tops of feet to the floor, find your feet and seat grounded, feet parallel and hip width apart.

QUALITIES: Acceptance, heart opening, enhances receptivity.

17. Half Shoulder Stand

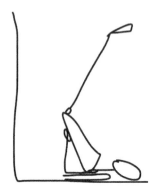

Fold a blanket in quarters and place one or more stacked blankets on the floor several feet from a wall, so that when your buttocks are near the wall you can lay on the blanket with the edge of the blanket level with the shoulders and the head on the floor. Bring the soles of the feet onto the wall, bent 90 degrees at the knee and support the low back with the palms, fingers pointing toward the ceiling. Elbows and upper arms are parallel to one another, tucked in even with the shoulders, and pressing down to the floor. Push the feet against the wall to move the hips away from the wall and lift one leg and then the other overhead with straight legs.

ALTERNATIVE: Proceed as above, but keep both feet on the wall, feet parallel to one another, pressing against the wall and lifting the hips. Another choice is **Legs Up The Wall Pose** (see 10, page 103): Begin by sitting next to the wall with the right hip touching the wall. Keeping as close to the wall as possible, lean back and swing the legs up the wall. You will end up lying on your back with the torso perpendicular to the wall and the legs together and extended toward the ceiling. You may be able to scoot toward the wall until the sit bones touch it, but it is fine to have the buttocks a few inches from the wall. If desired a folded blanket or bolster may be placed under the sacrum and low back, generally higher if you are more flexible, less high if you are stiffer.

QUALITIES: Cooling, contentment, finding a new perspective, intuition.

18. Camel Pose

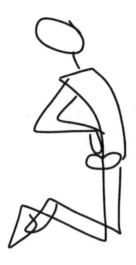

Come to a kneeling position with knees directly under the hips and feet directly behind the knees with toes curled under. A folded blanket can be placed under the knees for comfort. Engage the legs and navel and lift the sternum as the shoulders roll back and place the palms on the lower back with fingers pointing down. As the elbows move toward one another arch the upper back. The sternum may begin to face the ceiling, lengthening the front and back of the torso. Keep pressing the hips forward and pressing down with the feet and knees. If the pose is achieved easily, reach one hand and then the other on the heels, keeping the chin slightly tucked in.

ALTERNATIVE: Kneel with hips facing the wall and proceed as above, pressing the hips toward the wall, keeping palms supporting the lower back.

QUALITIES: Heart opening, encourages self-expression, energizes, enhances flexibility.

19. Boat Pose

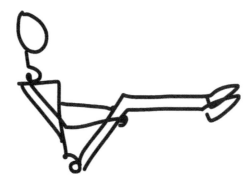

Begin seated on the floor with legs bent, feet on the floor, hip width apart. Bring hands behind the hips and lean back slightly lifting the sternum, taking care to not round the lower back. Then take the hands to the back of the knees with the arms straight. Continue to lean back as you come to the tips of the toes and engage the low belly. Hold there, and if it is comfortable to do so, lift one leg and the other until the shins are parallel to the ground, toes pointed. If this shape can be maintained, then release the hands and extend the arms parallel to the floor, arms straight, palms facing. Next, if possible, straighten one leg and then the other, toes pointed toward the place where the wall meets the ceiling, while the chin remains level with the floor and the sternum lifts.

ALTERNATIVE: Use a belt or yoga strap around the backs of the knees, clasping it on either side of the thighs, or use the strap at the insteps and straighten the legs with arms straight, maintaining alignment as above.

QUALITIES: Stress relieving, focusing, enhances concentration, improves confidence.

20. Reverse Table Pose/Staff Pose

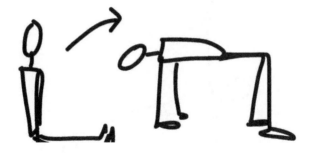

Begin in **Staff Pose**, seated on the floor with legs extended out in front, toes pointed toward the ceiling, legs engaged. Sit erect with palms on the floor next to the hips. Next, press the hands down and lift the knees to bring the soles of the feet to the floor. Press the soles of the feet and the hands as you engage the core and lift the hips to bring the torso level with the floor and knees directly over the ankles. Without moving the hands, tuck the chin and round the back to bring the seat back to the floor between the hands. Repeat.

ALTERNATIVE: Tabletop Pose/Child's Pose

If the movement described above is too strenuous you may begin **Tabletop Pose**: on hands and knees facing the floor, align the hands directly below the shoulders and the knees directly under the hips. Engage the navel and have the torso level with the floor. Then, keeping the hands right where they are, exhale and lower the seat toward the heels coming into Child's Pose (1, page 94) with arms extended. Moving with slow deep breaths, press down on the tops of feet and press the palms into the floor as you inhale back up to hands and knees. Repeat.

QUALITIES: Stability, steadiness, determination, adaptability.

21. Side Arm Balance

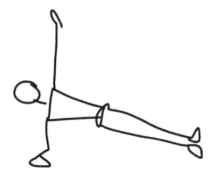

Begin in **Plank Pose** (see 15, page 108) and bring the weight into the right hand, turn the hips to the left and come to the outer edge of the right foot, stacking the left leg on top of the right and bringing the left hand to the left hip. Press down through the right palm, engage the core and lift the rotated hips toward the ceiling. Reach the left hand toward the ceiling with elbow straight and palm facing out if the balance is comfortable. Repeat on the opposite side.

ALTERNATIVES: Begin in **Plank Pose** and step the left foot halfway forward toward the hips, proceed as above with the left foot on the floor for support. Another choice is to begin instead in **Forearm Plank Pose**, where forearms are on the floor parallel to one another with the elbows directly under the shoulders and legs are extended with a straight line from the crown to the heels as in regular **Plank Pose** (see 15, page 108). Bring the weight onto the right arm and rotate the forearm so that it comes perpendicular to the line of the body. Rotate the hips so that the left hip stacks over the right and bring the left hand to the left hip. Stack the feet so the weight rests on the outer edge of the right foot and hips lift toward the ceiling. Place a block under the right hip if desired. Reach the left hand toward the ceiling with elbow straight and palm facing out if the balance is comfortable. Repeat on the opposite side.

QUALITIES: Strengthening, promotes balance, enhances confidence, integration.

22. Kundalini Crow Pose

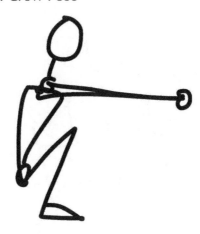

Begin by standing with feet greater than hip width apart with feet slightly turned out. Interlace the fingers with only the index fingers extended. Extend the arms parallel to the ground, arms straight. Bend the knees into a squat with the feet flat on the ground. Lean forward slightly; the ribcage will rest on the thighs. Gaze directly over the index fingers.

ALTERNATIVE: Begin as above, but instead of keeping the feet flat, allow the heels to lift and squat on the balls of the feet. Another choice is to allow the buttocks to touch a wall for steadiness. If squatting is not possible perform the pose seated in a chair.

QUALITIES: forgiveness, compassion, connection to nature, sincerity.

23. Squat Pose

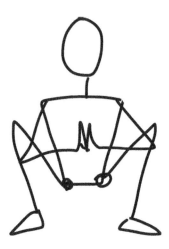

Begin in a standing position with feet wider than hip width and toes turned slightly out. Bring palms together at the heart in Anjali mudra (see 25, page 81), forearms parallel to the ground. Bend the knees deeply and lower the seat toward the floor. Bring the elbows inside the knees, broaden across the collarbones and lift the crown of the head and move shoulders away from the ears. Engage the low belly and avoid rounding the low back.

ALTERNATIVE: Proceed as above with a folded blanket supporting the heels and/or a block under the seat for support. Or, assume the pose with the back pressed against a wall. If squatting is impossible one can lie on the floor with the torso perpendicular to the wall, buttocks a few inches from the wall and the soles of the feet pressing onto the wall, greater than hip width with the toes turned out slightly.

QUALITIES: Stability, awareness, grounding, integration, cultivates patience.

24. Corpse Pose

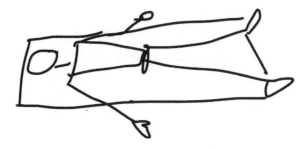

Begin by sitting on the floor with legs bent. Roll back until you are supporting yourself on your elbows. Lift the pelvis slightly and move it slightly toward the ankles. As you lower the pelvis, slightly drag the buttocks so that the lower spine is neutral as you straighten the legs. Feet fall out to the sides, relaxed. Next, lower the upper body to the floor, then slightly lift one shoulder and then the other, moving the shoulder blades more firmly on the back. Allow the arms to be long at the sides, palms up, slightly away from the body. Soften all the muscles of the body and come to stillness.

ALTERNATIVE: If the lower back is uncomfortable then place a bolster or folded blanket under the knees, and if the neck is uncomfortable place a thin layer of blanket under the head so that the forehead is parallel to the floor. If getting onto the floor is impossible then sit comfortably erect in a chair, with a pillow supporting the back and forearms on the thighs, palms facing up. Come to stillness.

QUALITIES: Calming, stress relieving, mood elevating, balancing.

25. Partner Chair Pose

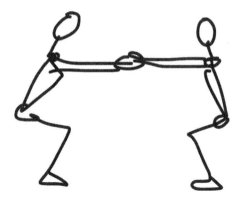

Begin with two people facing one another. Be sure the partners are willing to work together. Make sure both have performed Chair Pose. In **Chair Pose** feet are hip width and parallel to one another. The knees are bent, taking care to keep knees over the ankles, and the seat extends back, as if sitting in a chair, and spine remains straight. The hands can remain on the hips, or straight arms are extended overhead with shoulders relaxing away from the ears. The two people then face one another, spaced so that fingers touch with arms extended. Then both partners extend their arms out straight and parallel to the floor. They each clasp the other person's wrists and lean back slightly with straight spines to find full extension of the arms. Adjust the feet accordingly, with each person keeping feet hip width and parallel to one another. Maintaining the mutual tugging of the extended arms, partners should simultaneously bend the knees to come into Chair Pose, with thighs parallel to the floor.

ALTERNATIVE: Two people who have done Chair Pose individually and are willing to work together can come back to back. Interlace arms at the elbows. Keeping contact along the entire back body the two simultaneously bend the knees any amount, coming into Chair Pose.

QUALITIES: Trust,   strength,   compassion,   cooperation, interdependency.

26. Bridge Pose

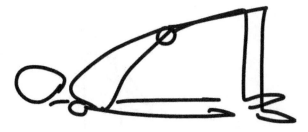

Begin by lying on the back with knees bent and feet directly under the knees, parallel to one another. Press evenly into the feet and strongly and slowly lift the hips. Roll one shoulder and then the other under the back, pressing the palms flat on the floor. Alternatively you may wish to clasp the hands beneath the raised buttocks, and push the hands towards the floor. Lengthen the back and engage the low belly. Shoulders move away from the ears, sternum lifts toward the chin. Chin remains neutral.

ALTERNATIVE: Half Bridge Pose
Begin as above, lying on the back with bent knees and feet directly under the knees, parallel to one another. Lift the hips enough to create a straight line from the knees to the shoulders. Place a block or other support under the pelvis at its lowest height. Extend the arms at the sides, palms down, pressing the entire arm to the floor.

QUALITIES: Heart opening, mental clarity, reduces anxiety, lifts mood.

27. Lunge Pose

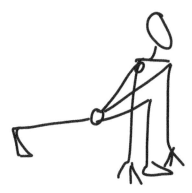

Begin in **Mountain Pose** (see 3, page 96). Fold forward with knees bent and bring the palms flat on the floor on either side of the feet. Take a long step back with the right foot, toes curled under and heel pressing back. Roll the shoulders back with arms straight and make sure the left knee is directly over the left ankle. Engage the right leg and level the hips. Come to fingertips and square the chest, looking forward. Breathe. Repeat on the opposite side OR if all goes well come to **High Lunge Pose**: Engage by pulling everything in toward the midline of the body and lift both arms overhead with palms facing and fingers extended. The head will be between the upper arms, gaze forward, chin parallel to the floor. Repeat on the opposite side.

ALTERNATIVE: As above, begin in **Mountain Pose** (see 3, page 96). Fold forward with knees bent and bring the palms flat on the floor on either side of the feet. Take a long step back with the right foot, toes curled under and heel pressing back. Roll the shoulders back with arms straight and make sure the left knee is directly over the left ankle. Engage the right leg and level the hips. Rest the gaze a few feet ahead on the floor and bring two stacked blocks or an armless chair to support the thigh of the forward leg. Another choice is to place a block under each hand.

QUALITIES: Enhances self-control, confidence, grounding, balance.

28. Seated Wide Leg Forward Bend

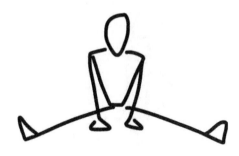

Begin seated on the edge of a folded blanket. Lift long through the spine and open the legs wide in a "V" shape with the toes pointing toward the ceiling. Place the palms down, shoulder width, on the floor in front of you. Hinge the body forward at the hips, keeping the spine extended, and walk the hands forward. Use the support of the arms to draw yourself gently forward. Bend the knees as needed.

ALTERNATIVE: Take the pose as above, but if low back rounds add several blankets under the hips for more height. Place a chair in front of you and instead of placing the hands on the floor, fold the arms and rest them on the chair. As you tip the body forward place the forehead on the arms and gently push the chair away.

QUALITIES: Stability, openness, self-reflection, calming.

29. Stork Pose

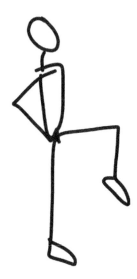

Begin in **Mountain Pose** (see 3, page 96). Bring hands to the hips and shift weight onto the right foot. Slowly lift your left leg until the thigh is parallel to the floor, knee at a 90-degree angle, toes pointing down. Engage the standing leg and press down through the heel. If balance is steady, bring arms straight out in front of the torso, parallel to the ground, shoulder width apart, palms facing. If steadiness continues, slowly bring arms upward, stopping where the shoulders are comfortable, or raising the arms so the upper arms are beside the ears. Repeat on the opposite side.

ALTERNATIVE: Begin in **Mountain Pose** (see 3, page 96), with the back of a chair arm's length away. Bring the hands, shoulder width apart, to the back of the chair. Shift weight onto the right foot. Slowly lift the left leg and lift the knee until the thigh is parallel to the floor, or as high as feels comfortable, allowing the toes to point toward the floor. Engage the standing leg and press the heel to the floor and press the palms to the top of the chair. Repeat on the opposite side.

QUALITIES: Inward focus, centeredness, balance, attentiveness.

30. Downward Facing Dog Pose

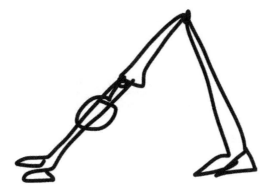

Begin in **Tabletop Pose**, with hands directly under shoulders and knees under hips. Curl the toes under and lift the hips, pushing down through the hands and all ten fingers. Bend knees slightly as needed and engage the thighs, rotating them inward as you reach the heels toward the floor. Lift the navel and lengthen the torso. Broaden across the chest, move the shoulder blades down the back and allow the head to relax between the upper arms, gazing toward the toes.

ALTERNATIVE: Modified Downward Dog Pose
Begin in **Mountain Pose** (see 3, page 96), facing a table, standing several feet away. Bring hands to the hips and hinge forward with a lengthened spine, as you reach forward to bring the palms face down on the table, sliding them forward until arms are straight. Bend the knees slightly as you engage the legs, internally rotating the thighs and lifting the navel. Roll the shoulder blades onto the back and broaden across the chest. Head is comfortably between the upper arms and the gaze is toward the floor. Engage the arms and press the palms onto the table.

QUALITIES: Improves self-confidence, reduces anxiety, provides a new perspective.

31. Forward Bend at Wall

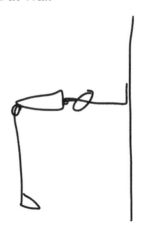

Begin in **Mountain Pose** (see 3, page 96), one foot away from and facing the wall. Place your palms against the wall a little above waist height, shoulder width apart. Walk the feet back as you press your hands to the wall until the body forms an "L" shape. The arms and torso form a straight line with the head between the upper arms, crown of the head facing the wall. Engage the legs with knees slightly bent, quadriceps lifting. Lift the navel as you lengthen the torso and engage the arms. Move the shoulders away from the ears as you broaden across the chest.

ALTERNATIVE: If there is discomfort or difficulty maintaining a flat back in an "L" shape then begin in **Mountain Pose** (see 3, page 96), one foot away from the wall and reach the hands several feet up the wall. Press the palms against the wall, shoulder width apart. Walk the feet away from the wall, and tip forward at the hips, allowing the torso to extend and incline toward the wall while engaged legs stay perpendicular to the floor with feet hip width apart and parallel to one another. Arms straighten as palms slide to a comfortable position and head is positioned between the upper arms. The navel lifts and shoulders relax away from the ears while the arms remain engaged.

QUALITIES: Comfort, stability, strength, introspection.

32. Dancer Pose

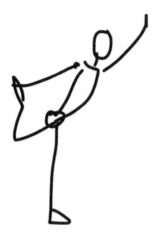

Begin in **Mountain Pose** (see 3, page 96). Bring hands to the hips and shift the weight to your right foot. Bending the knee, lift your left heel toward your seat and reach for the outer edge of your left foot with your left hand. Engage the standing leg and lift the navel as you push the left foot away from the buttock and into the left hand, keeping the knee and heel in line with the hip and keeping the torso relatively upright. If the balance is steady then sweep the right arm up next to the ear with palm facing inward. Repeat on the opposite side.

ALTERNATIVE: Stand in **Mountain Pose** (see 3, page 96), facing a wall, about two feet away from the wall. Reach the right arm up the wall and place the fingertips against the wall. Shift the weight to the right leg. Bend the left leg at the knee and either take hold of the outside of the foot with the left hand or use a yoga strap looped around the foot to pull the foot toward the body as you find balance. Another option is to take hold of the pant leg if that is more accessible than the foot or ankle. Keep the ankle, knee and the hip in line and then move the heel away from the seat so that it moves directly behind the left buttock, rather than out to the side. Tip forward slightly at the hips and move the fingertips up the wall as needed for steadiness. Repeat on the opposite side.

QUALITIES: Energizing, balance, concentration, centering.

Chapter 9

ART DIRECTIVES

The art directives used here are very simple. They are meant to be accessible and easy to follow with little instruction and without exotic materials. The Practice Chart (Table 5.1, pages 55–66) provides an example of how to put together a practice using a mudra meditation, a yoga pose and an art directive. Ideally, a person could do the practice daily, incorporating it into their routine, and therefore, the art making is designed to be accomplished quickly. If you wish to use the chart to create a group with a longer directive or you have the inclination to spend more time on the art-making portion, then the art making can be expanded. Experienced art therapists will understand that the materials and activity are selected for the effects they produce in most individuals. Like the mudras and yoga poses the art directives have certain qualities that are useful for further developing the intention that the practice is centered around.

This chapter will give directions for the directive and an idea of which qualities are evoked by including that form of art making into the practice. Use your experience and expertize to alter these according to your needs and desires. The instructions are purposefully open-ended so that the artist can modify freely. The framework for each project aligns with the intention established in that row of the chart. However, once you are experienced in matching the qualities found in the art making with those of the other components, you can create a practice from the starting point of the art directive you have in mind, and build accordingly.

The scope of this book does not cover all the clinical reasons for the choices of directives listed here. If you are an art therapist you will understand the clinical implications and modify accordingly. If you are adding art techniques to a practice as a yoga practitioner, please do not call it "art therapy" and do not attempt to address clinical concerns for which you do not have proper training. If you are not an art therapist the directives can simply be followed, keeping in mind the same guidelines with which you approach the other elements of this method. Everyone should remember that it is always advisable to experience the art-making technique yourself first if you plan to share it with others.

Directing versus teaching art

When we encounter art in our daily lives we are conditioned by our culture to make a judgment: "Do I like it or dislike it?", "Is this art good or bad?" If you were taking an art class, it would be appropriate to try to improve your skills; you would strive to make excellent work. In contrast, when following an art directive it is important to let go of that kind of judgment. Use the practice of meditation as a template for how to approach the art making. Let go of the natural tendency to control, and let your response to the directive flow. Meditation teaches us to witness rather than make value judgments. When you put aside the desire to make a "good" work of art then you are more likely to perceive the work objectively. Think of the activity as an opportunity to learn more about yourself. When it is time to discuss or process the art try to look at each project without judgment by making observations and asking questions.

PROCESSING THE ART MAKING

* Notice what it was like to respond to the directive.

* How did the materials feel?

* What might you do differently another time?

* Look at the finished piece. Put aside any judging tendencies and see what the image has to tell you.

* What do you notice?

* What questions come up?

* What have you learned?

Art Directives

1. GRATITUDE JOURNAL using images

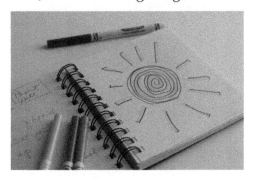

Begin with a blank book journal or any series of pages that are consistently sized and might be bound together upon completion. Any drawing material can be used. When it comes time to make art, think about what came up for you during the mudra meditation where you focused on "I am grateful for the support I have today." Create an image related to that gratitude. Take five minutes each day to record something that you are grateful for in the form of an image. After a week or more, look back through the images and notice what the cumulative effects are for you.

QUALITIES: Structured, projective, unifying, inward focusing.

2. Draw HOW YOU ARE FEELING right now

Begin with any drawing materials and any paper you have on hand. Take a moment to notice how you are feeling. Do you feel different than you did before you began the mudra meditation? Spend five minutes or more using color, line and/or image to create a drawing that shows anything you notice about how you are feeling right now.

QUALITIES: Expressive, sensory, enhancing perception, focusing.

3. Paint a MOUNTAIN and a VALLEY

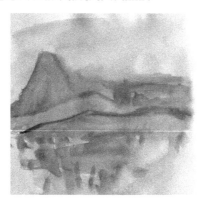

Begin with any size paper you like and drawing materials or paint. Use materials that you feel comfortable enough with to be able to complete a sketch in five to ten minutes. The directive is purposefully simple. Your mountain and valley might be different each time you make them.

QUALITIES: Projective, expressing conflict/meaning, balancing, grounding.

4. Do a CONTOUR DRAWING

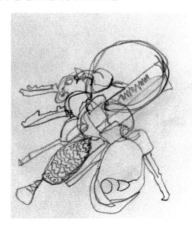

A drawing "from life" means that you look closely at an object, or person, and attempt to draw it being faithful to what you are looking at. It is not important if the result resembles the object you have chosen, the important part is to pay attention to what you are seeing. To do a contour drawing, use your eyes to trace each object, noticing the outlines rather than the details. Place the pencil on the paper and make your drawing with one continuous line and use your instincts to emphasize the object's essence. You may look from subject to the paper and back, but do not lift the pencil until you are finished. For a more sensory experience, try a "blind" contour drawing by using a continuous line to draw an object's outline without looking at the paper.

QUALITIES: Soothing, perception/observation enhanced, focusing.

5. Make a MANDALA

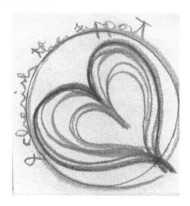

A mandala is simply a drawing inside a circle. The circle can be any size. Notice what it feels like to work within a circle.

QUALITIES: Freedom, containing, low structure, harmony, centering.

6. Create a collage using COLORED TAPE

Tape makes a wonderful collage material. It is a natural for creating abstract designs with minimal cutting and no glue. One suggestion for including this directive in a daily practice would be to use sturdy paper cut into squares. When the artist has completed a number of tape collages they can then be arranged as a "quilt" and different variations can be explored.

QUALITIES: Structured, sensory, potential for complexity, security.

7. Do a painting on a ROCK

Begin with a stone with a smooth surface, any size. Acrylic paint is recommended and it might be helpful to moisten the surface first, if the stone is porous. When the finished painting is dry it can be covered with several coats of clear acrylic varnish. Alternatively, one can draw on smooth stones with oil pastels for a nice effect.

QUALITIES: Simplicity, sensory, stability, soothing, grounding.

8. Make and decorate a SHIELD

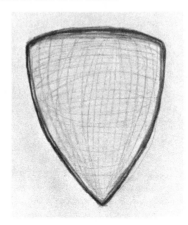

Cut sturdy paper into the shape of a shield, broad at the top and coming to a point at the bottom. The artist can imagine what qualities they possess that make them strong and capable and use those images as a starting point for their decoration. Drawing materials or cut paper and collage are good options for this directive.

QUALITIES: Containing, balancing, metaphorical, organizational skill, promotes self-confidence.

9. Create a STRENGTH QUILT

Using paper cut into squares create drawings depicting personal strengths. This project could be done over time as a daily practice, or as a single session. Plan the size of the squares and number of strengths accordingly. For example, a single session project could consist of four strength squares, each measuring 4" x 4" for an overall piece measuring 8" x 8". The artist can then rearrange the squares to find the most pleasing arrangement.

QUALITIES: Problem solving, expressive, finding meaning, promotes self-confidence.

10. Draw an INSIDE/OUTSIDE MANDALA

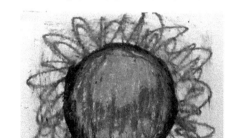

Directive 5 explains that a mandala is art created within a circular shape. For this directive begin with any size circle on paper leaving space for drawing around the circle. Using any drawing materials, create a drawing both within the circle and outside the circle.

QUALITIES: Soothing, containing, balancing, finding meaning, grounding.

11. Make a SELF-PORTRAIT

There are many approaches available for creating self-portraits. You can work from memory, or use a mirror to take a representational approach. Drawing materials, paint or even clay could be appropriate, keeping in mind the time each material demands. Another approach is to depict the "self" as an animal or object. Alternatively, you could brainstorm all the things that make you YOU and then create a magazine collage.

QUALITIES: Observation, perception, expressive, self-perception, self-acceptance.

12. Do an INNER VOICE project

In this directive the preceding meditation may be important for generating imagery. The artist asks, "What is my inner voice like?"

and answers this question using art materials. It might be nice to provide fabrics for a texture collage, although any material can work for this directive.

QUALITIES: Sensory, balancing, unifying, expressive, self-perception, stimulating.

13. Create a BODY MAP

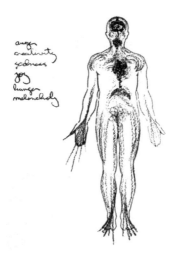

Body outlines can be printed for free from the internet. Here again, the meditation portion of the practice can be used to inform this art directive. The artist creates a list of feelings or the therapist guides the participant to notice where in the body different emotions are found. The artist can then create a personal color code for their feelings and use the corresponding colors to fill in the space of their body-map outline. This project can be greatly expanded by an experienced art therapist. Some clients will find it rewarding to be guided through a full body tracing and use paint or other materials to show where emotions occur in the body.

QUALITIES: Restrictive, expressive, harmony, organization, self-reflection.

14. Create a STRENGTHS COLLAGE

In this project cut-out magazine or newspaper photos are glued to paper. The artist chooses and arranges images to show their personal strengths.

QUALITIES: Making meaning, metaphor, containing, self-perception, self-confidence.

15. Make IMAGES of FEELINGS

Make a list of feelings. Begin with a stack of paper and have watercolors or other paint available. Working quickly, perhaps allowing two or three minutes per page, depict each word using color, line and texture.

QUALITIES: Fluency, metaphorical, perception, expressive, self-reflection.

16. Make BUBBLE PRINTS

Watercolor paper is best, but any paper will do. Combine a tablespoon of dish soap with water in a tray. Add liquid watercolor or diluted acrylic paint and swirl the mixture. Use a straw to blow bubbles and then lay the paper over the bubbles to create a print.

QUALITIES: Simplicity, soothing, fluidity, balancing, acceptance.

17. Create an INSIDE/OUTSIDE BOX

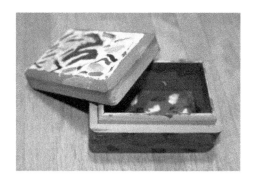

Ideally, begin with a box with a lid that has a solid color on the inside and the outside. A smaller box may be more manageable in a shorter time period. Then, using any materials that are comfortable to you, decorate the box. Collage, paint or oil pastels are all good options. On the outside, in whatever way you wish, show what you are like on the outside. On the inside of the box, show what you keep inside.

QUALITIES: Structured, metaphorical, projective, self-perception, self-reflection.

18. Respond to a FAMOUS WORK OF ART

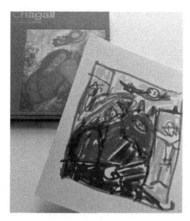

Begin with a well-known work of art, printed from the internet, or found in a book or on a postcard. Using any material, make your interpretation of the piece. This cannot be done incorrectly; it could mean incorporating the reproduction in the piece, drawing a likeness, or showing what it is that attracts you to it.

QUALITIES: Problem solving, enhancing perception, stimulating, acceptance, self-expression.

19. Make a CALMING LANDSCAPE

Begin with an art material that provides a variety of colors, or the opportunity to mix colors. Choose or create colors that you find soothing and make a landscape. Any size paper held horizontally is appropriate for your imaginary landscape.

QUALITIES: Soothing, containing, fluid, narrative, focusing.

20. Make APPRECIATION CARDS

This activity may be done with two or more people. Begin with sturdy paper, folded in half like a greeting card; one for each person. First, write your name on the back of the card. Next pass the card to the person on your right. Each time you receive a card look at the name on the back and with color, words or images make a visual message of appreciation for the original cardholder. The cards are complete when you receive your original card, full of messages from the other group members. Alternatively, create a card for someone, showing what you appreciate about him or her. The card does not necessarily have to be delivered, or even created for someone still living, the focus here is on expressing appreciation.

QUALITIES: Perception, harmony, expressive, balancing, adaptability.

21. Make a picture of POSITIVE THINGS

Using art materials that you enjoy, make a picture showing all the positive things in your life. This project can work well with magazine collage, using found images as inspiration or symbolic representation of positive aspects of your life.

QUALITIES: Symbolic, narrative, unifying, expressive, balancing.

22. Create a BOX OF VALUES

Think about what it is you value. Use a box with a lid and decorate the outside with magazine collage images that represent you. Fill the box with words, either cut from magazines, or written on paper, representing what you value most.

QUALITIES: Containing, complex, organization, self-expressive, sincerity.

23. Use a FOUND OBJECT as a PAINTBRUSH

Create a painting on watercolor paper or canvas board using tempera or acrylic paint. Instead of using a paintbrush do the painting with a found object. You may wish to assemble a few objects and experiment.

QUALITIES: Stimulating, problem solving, expressive, provides a new perspective, enhances perception.

24. Create an image of HOME

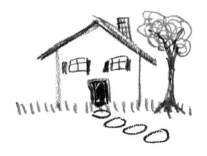

Begin with your favorite 2D or 3D materials and create an image of what "home" means to you.

QUALITIES: Projective, metaphorical, problem solving, expressive, balancing.

25. WORK COLLABORATIVELY

Begin by finding a partner willing to create a work of art with you. Together, make decisions about materials and how to proceed. With a sense of play, work together to make a piece of art.

QUALITIES: Provides a new perspective, problem solving, unifying, stimulating, promotes cooperation.

26. Make a FUTURE SELF-PORTRAIT

Imagine what qualities you would like to cultivate in the future. In whatever way you wish, and with any materials, show your ideas for your future self.

QUALITIES: Expressive, problem solving, projective, symbolic, self-perceptive.

27. Make a BLINDFOLD DRAWING

Let go of the idea of a beautiful product. Focus on the act of drawing. Close your eyes or place a blindfold over the eyes and do a drawing from your imagination without looking. Any drawing materials may be used.

QUALITIES: Provides a new perspective, stimulating, unifying, freeing, promotes self-control.

28. Create an ECCENTRIC INVENTION

An invention is a solution to a problem. What problem would you like to solve? Using your wildest imagination, create a drawing solving the problem in any way at all. Limit the materials to paper and pencil or colored pencils.

QUALITIES: Problem solving, perception, active, provides a new perspective, metaphorical.

29. Create ART FOR OTHERS

Using art materials that are comfortable for you, create a piece of art with another person or a group in mind. When you are finished, give the piece to the intended recipient.

QUALITIES: Expressive, stimulating, provides a new perspective, problem solving, compassion.

30. Make a SCRIBBLE DRAWING

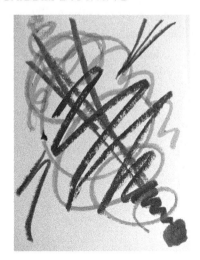

Begin with paper and drawing materials. Make a scribble. Take a moment to see what your scribble looks like and turn it into a drawing. You may want to make several scribbles on a single sheet of paper. Alternatively, you can make scribble drawings with a partner. You make a scribble for the other person to turn into a drawing and then trade roles, repeating until the page is filled.

QUALITIES: Freeing, soothing, expressing conflict, making meaning, provides a new perspective.

31. SEW A PILLOW

Begin with two rectangular pieces of felt. You will also need embroidery thread or floss, a darning needle and polyester fluff for stuffing. To connect the two pieces of felt, sew with a simple whipstitch around three edges. Fill the shape with fluff and then complete the stitching. Choices may be limited to various colors for the felt and stitching, or the felt could be painted with acrylic paint, or decorated with fabric markers.

QUALITIES: Soothing, containing, textural, metaphorical.

32. Make a BIG DRAWING

Tape a few feet of butcher paper to the wall. Choose a soft or fluid material that can cover a lot of ground, charcoal, pastel, oil pastel or paint. Make a picture using the whole paper. Alternatively, several smaller sheets of paper could be taped together from the back and be approached in the same manner.

QUALITIES: Active, freeing, expressive, perception enhanced.

Chapter 10

STRUCTURING SESSIONS

Now that all the pieces are in place, readers might begin to think about how to structure a session. The Intention Centered Yoga and Art Therapy Method works well for work with individuals or groups. In either case, the best approach is to stay flexible and attuned to the needs of those with whom you are working. The amounts of yoga, meditation and art can be dialled up or down according to your needs and inclinations. Your experience and intuition are your best guides. It is important to notice, as you begin to share the practice, that not only do the effects of the intention and all its permutations accumulate across the session but there is also a cumulative effect for individuals and group members, particularly when the sequence takes on the aspect of ritual.

Sessions for individuals

Let's begin with planning a session for an individual. The initial determination is to find out if the person is open to working with a combination of yoga and art. Please disclose what training you have and what has motivated you to suggest this method for this particular person. As you proceed, continue to work together in the creation of the ideal approach for each individual. Together you can come up with the concern you wish to address or the positive quality that you wish to promote in each session. This could emerge as a result of an initial consultation, or organically in the course of a normal session.

The focus can also be determined more spontaneously after a brief discussion or after a reflective meditation. An appropriate starting point from which to develop a structure is the positive quality which will help form an intention. With clinician support, the client creates a positive statement in the present tense that becomes their intention. If this is difficult for the person, the intention appearing in the chart, or one modified by the clinician, might be suggested and used. Or, the client may be given an intention from the chart to modify as they wish, until both clinician and client are satisfied. Ideally, the client will have an "ah-ha" moment where the intention's message and tone resonate in a way that feels right.

The next step is to find a mudra that is comfortable for the client to hold for several minutes. The clinician can use the mudra suggested by the chart or substitute one with similar qualities from the explanations in Chapter 6. The person should be able to hold the mudra with a sense of ease. At this point the clinician offers a chance to practice meditation combining the mudra with the silent repetition of the intention. One way to begin the meditation is for the clinician to sit opposite the client, either on the floor in a comfortable cross-legged position, or in chairs, with feet flat on the floor. Alternatively, client and clinician can be seated opposite one another at a table, chairs pulled slightly away so that the hands and arms can rest freely as needed, and with feet on the floor. Props may be useful here. If seated on the floor, sitting up on a folded blanket or block can be useful, and sitting against a wall may help to achieve a long, erect spine without effort. When seated in a chair, if the feet do not reach the floor comfortably then place a support under the feet, perhaps thin blocks or several books. If a person has long legs then a cushion or blanket on the seat of the chair can create a comfortable flat-footed position. Another useful suggestion is to place a cushion between the clients back and the back of the chair to encourage erect posture.

Ask the client to sit in such a way that their seat and feet feel a grounded connection with the floor or chair. They should stretch the spine long and align the hips, shoulders and ears directly over one another. Once the mudra is assumed, the client should relax the shoulder blades down the back and either rest a soft gaze at a spot on the floor or table, or gently close the eyes. The clinician can then guide the client to take one to three deep cleansing breaths. A deep cleansing breath is a long inhale through the nose and an exhale through the mouth, perhaps with a sound or a sigh. Then, speaking aloud, the client and clinician together may repeat the intention from one to three times, coordinating the phrasing with the inhale and the exhale. The clinician then guides the client to continue, repeating the intention silently for one to three minutes (or longer for an experienced meditator). The clinician then asks the client to gently open the eyes, release the mudra and take a deep cleansing breath. Please note that the clinician should work with eyes open throughout the practice, observing the client and insuring that comfort is maintained.

The clinician will then offer a yoga pose or series of yoga poses to the client. A good starting point is either Mountain Pose (see 3, page 96) or Seated Mountain Pose. This pose establishes a foundation where the client can get a sense of their body and breath. From Mountain Pose, the person can move into any of the other poses with awareness of body and breath. A single pose, practiced with awareness, can be sufficient for establishing the aspect of the intention that is communicated through the manipulation of the body. If you wish to offer more poses you may consult the descriptions (see yoga poses in Chapter 8) to find the closely related poses. In each pose, guide the duration of the pose by tracking the breath. Breath should be strong and steady with inhale and exhale occurring through the nose. The pose can be held steadily for three to five breaths or up to a minute or more. Poses that have two sides should be held equally on each side. The clinician can speak aloud for guidance; for example, "Hold the pose for three breaths; inhale… exhale…inhale…exhale…inhale…exhale…" Complete the yoga pose part of the session by returning to Mountain Pose and taking a deep cleansing breath.

Now, with as smooth a transition as possible, move to the art materials. Ideally, the materials are readily at hand and the client can move into art making while maintaining the quiet focus established from the practice of meditation and yoga. The client spends time exploring the art directive. Throughout the practice it may be important to remind the client to release any tendency to judge, and instead observe and ask questions. This can happen at every stage, but it is especially important in the verbal processing of the art.

The discussion that follows the art making is a wonderful way to bring the practice back to the conscious mind. Please allow time for the artist to speak about their process. The discussion may relate back to the intention or simply be led by observations. The breakdown of timing depends greatly on the individual's comfort level and inclinations as well as the clinician's personal and clinical choices.

50-MINUTE SEQUENCE FOR AN INDIVIDUAL SESSION

1. (10 mins) Together the client and clinician develop an intention in response to the client's concern.

2. (5 mins) The client assumes a mudra and meditates using the intention as a mantra.

3. (10 mins) Client comes into Mountain Pose for 1 breath; then is guided through a yoga pose, 5 breaths (or more) on the left, 5 breaths on the right. Client ends in Mountain Pose taking a deep cleansing breath.

4. (20 mins) The client follows the art directive.

5. (5 mins) Together the client and clinician process the artwork.

Self-guided practice

Some clinicians like to give the client homework to continue the effects of the session throughout the week. Yoga and art can be practiced daily. Repeating the same sequence reinforces the intention and allows the client to build strengths within the practice. The homework might be to perform a short version of the practice they learned in the session.

A person could also use this book and the Practice Chart for Intention Centered Yoga and Art to find a self-guided practice of their own. In this case, the duration of each section can be fairly even, as in the daily practice above. Another way to use the practice is to decide which section resonates the most for you and expand that section, keeping the balance of the sections evenly timed with one another.

AN EXAMPLE OF A DAILY YOGA AND ART PRACTICE

1. (5 mins) Mudra meditation, using an intention as a mantra.

2. (5 mins) Yoga pose practice. Come into Mountain Pose for 1 breath, then move into pose and take 3 breaths left and right or 5 breaths of a single posture.

3. (5 mins) Create a simple version of the art directive.

4. Keep a written journal to reflect on the process, if desired.

Group sessions

Yoga and art practice lends itself well to group facilitation. The group format can mirror the individual structure. It can also grow or condense in any area as necessary. The structure is flexible as long as the intention remains the focus. When you are planning a group session begin by thinking about the needs of the group. What is an overriding concern at this time? What positive attribute would you like the group to cultivate? The answers to these questions will help you to concentrate on a theme or intention. It works best if the clinician has a concern in mind, but be prepared to respond to input from the group. In some cases the group will help to form an intention that feels right for those in attendance. It is best to begin the group by developing an intention and then proceed from there. A verbal check-in is a way of taking the temperature of the group and establishing a direction from which an intention can be created. An essential element for working with groups is consistency. The structure that the facilitator finds comfortable should be repeated each time the group meets. The sequence then becomes a ritual for the group. The clinician may include several aspects of ritual in the structure. For example, one way to anchor the practice is to always begin the meditation with three long deep breaths.

Art therapists might be constrained by the necessity of preparation work before an art group. If the art activity is the priority then you will decide on the concern you wish to address in that session and choose an art directive. Introduce the theme that is suggested by the art directive and use the client input to finalize an intention. Then, a brief mudra meditation and yoga pose practice can prepare the group for engagement in the art making.

A yoga practitioner might choose to extend the yoga-based parts of the structure and keep the art section relatively brief. The important consideration here is to keep the intention in mind and shape the practice accordingly. Different groups will have different requirements and needs. Create the structure that suits the group and maintain consistency to enhance the security of the group, whether yoga- or art-based.

The order of the sections could also shift if the facilitator finds a different sequence more appropriate. For example, some clients might benefit from equal time for yoga and art. In that case, it would make sense to put together a yoga sequence, which would be introduced after establishing an intention. The mudra meditation

STRUCTURING SESSIONS   149

could then happen after the poses and act as a transition to the art-making time. Some practitioners prefer to introduce the art first and for certain populations; this can work well too. The priority is to allow the intention to be echoed in various ways while maintaining a secure and positive experience for all the group members.

90-MINUTE STRUCTURE FOR AN ART-BASED GROUP

1. (5 mins) Check-in and develop an intention.

2. (5 mins) Mudra meditation using the intention: Follow an established ritual like beginning with 3 deep cleansing breaths. Assume the mudra. Speak the intention together aloud 3 times. Repeat the intention silently 1 time. Take 1 deep cleansing breath.

3. (10 mins) Yoga pose practice: Come to Mountain Pose; take 3 breaths. Move into the pose suggested in the chart; take 5 breaths or 3 breaths on each side, right and left. Optional: Continue practice by choosing related poses and holding for 3 to 5 breaths. Come back to Mountain Pose. Return to the mudra introduced in the beginning. Take a deep cleansing breath.

4. (40 mins) Art directive.

5. (5 mins) Clean up and clear the space.

6. (20 mins) Verbal processing of artwork.

7. (5 mins) Verbal check-out.

A case study

A case study is useful to show how convenient it is to have a chart or system to put together the various elements of the Intention Centered Yoga and Art Practice. The chart is handy but always remember that the vital element in the mix is to make the practice your own, whether you are practicing for yourself, instructing as a yoga teacher or offering yoga to support an art therapy practice. The following case study looks at an individual's experience in an art-based group structured around the 90-minute format suggested above. The subject of the case study is a composite portrait of a typical group member in a substance abuse treatment program.

> Harold, a 50-year-old African American male, regularly attended a yoga and art therapy group for approximately five months. The group was conducted in a non-profit residential substance abuse rehabilitation facility in a metropolitan area, serving men of diverse backgrounds. Criteria for inclusion in the group were substance abuse complicated by a significant history of trauma. Harold struggled with substance abuse, particularly abuse of alcohol, and he was diagnosed with advanced chronic obstructive pulmonary disease (COPD). He was referred to the group because of a history of physical and emotional abuse in his family of origin. Harold exhibited symptoms of trauma such as a limited range of emotional expression and chronic low-level depression. Harold was formerly a commercial artist but had not worked for several years due to substance abuse and health concerns.

> Harold was present for a weekly group session, which took place midway in the course of his treatment. At this point, Harold generally arrived on time, in contrast to earlier weeks when someone would often have to go find him and remind him about the group. Each group began with a check-in, an opportunity for the facilitator to introduce an idea for the day's intention and assess the group's needs. Check-in this day was to name a feeling that they had experienced recently. Harold appeared distracted and had to hunt to come up with a feeling. Harold often exhibited a common symptom of trauma where restless agitation replaces the person's ability to remain focused and attentive to what is happening in the present. He eventually said that he felt "frustrated." A list of feeling words was created from

each person's contribution. Because of the group's response, the facilitator decided that the idea of addressing the group's agitation, by cultivating serenity (see no. 15 on the chart) was an appropriate theme for the day. An experience of serenity supports the chance to regain self-control and the ability to make choices rather than merely reacting to daily occurrences.

The group was asked to find their feet on the floor, to feel their seat in their chairs and then to lift the top of their heads, extending their spines. They went on to take several deep, cleansing breaths. Breathing together brings the group together, helps them to be present in the room and shift their attention away from the concerns of the day. Harold organized himself in his chair and although deep breathing was not apparent, the habitual bouncing of his leg calmed and his eyes closed. Earlier in the course of the group, Harold's eyes would remain open at this point in the session. While he always behaved respectfully, his body did not always respond readily; typically, nervous habits would continue. It seemed that at this point in the group he had adjusted to the routine. The repetition of the practice had made it possible for Harold to begin to receive its benefits.

Next, Jalashaya mudra (no. 15 on the chart) was introduced. This mudra suggests calming, cooling, soothing and balancing. The men enjoyed the challenge of creating the hand gesture and Harold's shoulders visibly lowered when the group were encouraged to relax their shoulders. An intention was suggested to the group and Harold repeated it aloud, three times, "As I breathe, I experience serenity." As the group repeated the intention silently, a sense of serenity became apparent in the room. Harold remained calm during the short meditation and was attentive, responding immediately when asked to come to a standing position. The room was small, and the group members' physical abilities varied widely. The facilitator chose Mountain Pose (no. 3 on the chart) as a replacement for Plank Pose (no. 15 on the chart), which would not be practical in this case. Mountain Pose has some of the same qualities as Plank Pose, promoting inner strength, stabilization and serenity. Because the group was accustomed to yoga practice and the time was not too tight, a half Sun Salute was added to the sequence. Half Sun Salute both reinforced the qualities of the mudra and the initial yoga pose while the movement invigorated the group, preparing them for activity.

For the Half Sun Salute sequence the group was instructed to begin in Mountain Pose. On the inhale they raised their hands above their heads for Extended Mountain Pose. On the exhale they moved into Forward Bend, folding over their legs any amount. On the next inhalation they were asked to bend their knees slightly and roll through the spine back up to Mountain Pose. Two repetitions were enough for Harold to establish and maintain his physical and mental focus. The unrushed and gentle quality of his movements revealed the qualities the yoga practice was meant to promote: stability, strength, willpower. The group returned to Jalashaya mudra, this time finding it with ease. Together the group took a long, deep breath. A final repetition of the intention closed the yoga portion of the session.

The group moved quietly into the art-making directive. The attentiveness of the group was apparent as the facilitator explained that each person would create a painting for each of the feeling words that were listed during check-in. Eight members each had identified a word to answer the question "How are you feeling right now?" The project suggested in the chart (no. 15) where an individual might have created a single painting was expanded upon here. Eight 6" x 9" sheets of watercolor paper and a set of watercolors were offered to each group member. They wrote a word from the list on the back of each sheet and then proceeded to paint an expression of each feeling.

Harold made eight paintings, carefully altering line, color, shape and technique to express the qualities of different emotions. The time was limited for each emotion so that the group would have time to process their reactions to the directive. Harold had no trouble regulating the timing and finding varied means of expression descriptive of each emotion on the list. All the group members were eager to share their paintings. The room was full of paintings. Each person arranged their paintings and cleaned up the materials. Group members took turns presenting their work and were able to find similarities and differences in their approach to and execution of the directive. Group members noticed that Harold's work showed a range of approach: some pieces were dense with marks, others more fluid and sparse. With Harold's work, as well as that of others, participants could begin to guess which painting was made for each emotion. The group ended with a check-out where group members were asked to say one thing that they learned about themselves in the course of the day's session. Harold said that he was amazed that he could come into the room distracted and frustrated only to find that the hour and a half flew by and he did not want to leave because he was feeling so good.

Harold's experience in this group shows the integrated effects of yoga and art therapy. Treatment goals for the group were addressed throughout the session. Positive response to the group was so apparent that group members were able to identify nuanced emotional information comfortably and demonstrate a measure of control. Harold's response to this session was in keeping with his increasing ability to relate to other group members, make positive choices, remain focused and express a range of emotions.

Harold left the program several weeks later. At that time he appeared healthier and although his condition was still quite serious, coughing and other symptoms of his COPD had apparently improved. At that point, Harold was able to express himself with a range of emotion, especially evident in the enthusiasm he demonstrated for the future and the optimism expressed in regard to his sobriety.

Chapter 11

OTHER CONSIDERATIONS

This book has attempted to offer a simple and gentle means of practicing yoga and art techniques with mindfulness and attention to one's own physical and mental responses. Intention Centered Yoga and Art is an appropriate method for anyone to use to combine the practice of yoga with art making to seek balance and healing. The system also links beautifully with professional clinical practices, provided one is mindful of the ethical considerations in doing so.

Scope of practice

Trained professionals can use the Practice Chart in this book to offer art and yoga techniques that will empower clients to develop a personal healing practice in conjunction with their treatment. Art therapists wishing to make yoga practices a part of their treatment planning would be advised to obtain yoga training. Likewise, yoga teachers or yoga therapists who wish to use art therapy techniques to address mental health issues with their students must consider art therapy training. Valid concerns exist in regard to psychotherapists offering yoga-based practices to their clients without yoga training. Likewise, there is apprehension among professionals about yoga teachers and yoga therapists attempting to address mental health issues without in-depth mental health training (Weintraub 2013).

Yoga teachers, yoga therapists, psychotherapists and art therapists must decide what lies within their scope of practice. To combine modalities ethically, practitioners should first make clear to their clients what training they have completed. They should have a clear understanding of their role, and their limits in respect to confidentiality before combining modalities in treatment of any kind (Furman 2013). Today, with so many approaches to therapy of all kinds, practitioners must consider what constitutes their scope of practice. Sometimes a governing body such a licensing board enumerates requirements for education and training and defines exactly what a professional person is permitted to practice. If no such governing body exists in your locale for your area of expertise there is still a limit to the range of services you can provide responsibly. Please seek proper supervision if you have questions about what constitutes an ethical scope of practice. Combining modalities is most effective if the practitioner has training in each element they choose to combine with their primary practice.

In combining yoga with art therapy it is important to maintain integrity by being clear about treatment and boundaries. Art therapists are meant to treat cases for which their training qualifies them. They observe confidentiality and explain the expectations of the therapist–client relationship at the outset of any treatment. This means that an art therapist may use yoga techniques in support of their art psychotherapy, not to replace the therapy for which they are trained and possibly licensed to provide. It also means that they avoid dual relationships.

Yoga

Yoga has become ubiquitous in the West. As wonderful as it is to have easy access to yoga classes, it is possible that its proliferation has outstripped its professional oversight. The Yoga Alliance, in the case of yoga teachers and the International Association of Yoga Therapists, are both attempting to address this problem. Yoga is indeed for everyone, but every approach is not for everyone. Finding the correct approach involves seeking appropriate guidance.

Traditionally yoga was exclusively practiced one on one, so that the teacher, or guru, would carefully monitor the student's responses to every aspect of the practice. New poses, breathing techniques or meditations were suggested, as the student was ready. Part of that readiness was the student's increasing ability to self-monitor the reactions they were experiencing in the body and mind. Thus, learning "yoga" was akin to working with a holistically minded therapist today.

As yoga was introduced to Western practitioners, traditional yoga was modified to suit the Western lifestyle. Now, many students can be accommodated in large classes where the student is expected to modify their practice for themselves and the teacher teaches a fixed level and approach. The Western tendency toward self-directed autonomy is apparent in this development. The approach recommended in this book is closer to the traditional guru–student relationship. Keep in mind that the guru had also worked for many years with his own guru and therefore had in-depth training that he learned and assimilated through his own daily practice. A guru would be thoroughly familiar with any techniques he would teach, as well as being intimately familiar with the effects of the practices. The question of scope of practice would not occur under such circumstances. Anyone sharing yoga practices with others should thoroughly understand what they are teaching through personal practice and experience and should not attempt to address any conditions for which they do not have professional training.

Yoga therapy

Like art therapists, yoga therapists may face a scope of practice quandary. Although yoga therapy is not yet licensed, the profession is moving toward regulation. Yoga therapy is beginning to emerge as a separate profession from yoga teaching with schools becoming accredited and standards being established (IAYT 2014). However, the range of what may be called yoga therapy practice is still quite broad and practitioners should be careful about what they consider their scope of practice, particularly in regard to psychotherapeutic techniques. In this book, art directives are suggested, however, please understand that their application in the context of psychotherapy is only safely and ethically practiced with art therapy training. Just as art therapists should not use yoga therapeutically without training and supervision, the same is true for yoga therapists using art techniques. Art can be used in support of yoga therapy but may not be called art therapy or be practiced as such without the graduate level training discussed above.

Guidelines for adding yoga to art therapy practice

The most important advice for those offering yoga and art is to try out the technique you intend to use. While you are performing the practice, keep the person or group in mind before you work with them directly. This will give you invaluable insight into any pitfalls that might arise and then you can modify your offerings before the session. Of course, the experience of the effects and the ability to assimilate them will vary greatly.

Exercising caution while practicing yoga is advised for everyone. In sharing Intention Centered Yoga and Art as a clinician, experience with yoga practice cannot be overemphasized. You will be able to offer yoga techniques safely and effectively if you understand from your own experience what it is like to create poses, mudras and meditations in your own mind and body. Your experience with looking within and feeling the effects of breath, movement and contemplation will allow you to observe both the similar and different effects in other people. Additionally, be careful about the use of touch. In the Practice Chart for Intention Centered Yoga and Art (Table 5.1) the poses do not require manual adjustment. If you wish to communicate through the use of touch, please be aware of applicable laws governing the use of touch in therapy. It is always best for yoga teachers and therapists to consider if the use of touch is essential and truly in the client's best interest. If so, be sure to ask before placing hands on another person and be prepared to respect their wishes. Be certain that your touch is both emotionally supportive and physically stabilizing (Parker 2013).

Inevitably, a group or individual will be resistant to the use of yoga poses. Particularly in a group situation remind the members that participation is optional. The abstaining group members are encouraged to remain respectful and will generally receive benefits from simply being present in the group. During each session everyone is invited to try. Often, resistant folks will eventually find themselves comfortable enough to give it a go. These practices are completely unrelated to the competitive manner in which most Westerners attempt almost any physical endeavor. Be vigilant about noticing this tendency first in yourself and then in any person with whom you are working.

Do be aware that not all those who attempt yoga poses and other techniques are in tune with the reactions present in their bodies and minds. You will need to closely monitor breathing, facial expression and bodily tension. If a person is holding their breath, grimacing or making gripping actions with any parts of their body (jaw, fists, shoulders, etc.) take note and suggest a modification or end the practice. Often, yoga teachers will demonstrate poses and meditation techniques by simultaneously practicing along with the student/s. If you would like to demonstrate, please do so by asking the student or client to observe your actions first, so that when they perform the action you are free to observe. Do not close your eyes even during meditation. You must discreetly watch what is going on for the individual or group at all times.

Physical cautions

The practices suggested in this book are gentle and meant to be practiced without any experience of pain. Pain, of course, is subjective. If people move their bodies and breathe in novel ways they may experience sensations that are unfamiliar. You might ask your students or clients to discriminate carefully between sensation and pain. Pain should always be avoided. However, sensation may be explored. Sensation is to be experienced without judgment. It is possible to avoid the tendency to label sensation as "good" or "bad" if the focus remains on the breath. "Breathing into" sensation is encouraged as a way of tolerating the novelty and isolating the experience separate from the "story" or meaning that might be given to the sensation. Instruct the student to inhale deeply and then to imagine that their exhale can travel to the area of sensation and help the muscles and tissue relax and release into the position. Several breaths using this evaluation method can help the person decide whether to move away from strong sensation that might cause pain, or deeper into the experience of sensation in order to learn more about the effects the position might have on the body and mind.

Also, please defer to the advice of the student or client's physician in every case. Those with high blood pressure or eye conditions should not perform poses where the head is below the heart without their doctor's permission. If any other health conditions exist ask the client to check with their physician before performing any yoga techniques.

Trauma history

When practicing Intention Centered Yoga and Art it is necessary to develop sensitivity toward those who may have a history of trauma. Both yoga therapy and art therapy have specialized training available for those who wish to work with trauma survivors. It is important to keep in mind that any person you may find yourself working with could have a trauma history that has not been disclosed. Symptoms could inadvertently be triggered by yoga or art practices. At the same time, research is proving that both yoga- and art-based interventions can be highly effective in trauma treatment if trauma-sensitive approaches are followed. These findings are based on the fact that "our minds can be 'slippery'; people can sometimes engage in talk therapy for years and never access important aspects of their inner experience" (Emerson and Hopper 2011, p.24). The reconstruction of the self after trauma needs to be experienced by the body and the mind together (Dayton 2000).

Trauma symptoms may be expressed in the form of flashbacks, dissociation, anxiety and limited emotional range, to name a few. Feedback from the client and your observations can help you to become sensitive to these conditions. In general, yoga- and art-based approaches help to build a connection to the self that can begin to alleviate these symptoms. Offering choices, cultivating the ability to remain present and grounded, and encouraging the observation of inner and outer experience are the features of this book's practices that are also important elements of trauma sensitivity. Applying these concepts with mindfulness will create the structure and safety that can be groundwork for healing.

Guidelines for adding art to yoga therapy practice

The same advice that was presented to art therapists offering yoga applies to yoga teachers offering art to students, clients or groups. Try out the technique you intend to use. While you are making art, keep the person or group in mind before you work with them directly. Imagine that the issue or concern affects you and take note of the project's effects. Familiarity with the materials and processes will inform you about how the project will be received. There are many variables in each project that can be altered to suit your needs. Sometimes a very simple, quick art endeavor is appropriate. At other times you may wish to challenge a person or group with a more intricate and time-consuming directive.

Art-making considerations

Some aspects of art making to consider are timing, materials, paper/project size, complexity, experience level of participant/s and motor skill levels. Art therapists are skilled in considering these components in art-based groups. The projects recommended in the Practice Chart for Intention Centered Yoga and Art have been selected to both address the stated concern and to dovetail with the effects of the yoga, which will likely precede the art making. The following explanations may help you to adjust the directives to your needs with insight and confidence.

Timing

Timing is an important aspect of the art project. The position of art making at the end of the chart is purposeful. Usually the physical practices allow the participant to become receptive to trying new things and to working with awareness. In some instances it may be appropriate to place art making at the beginning of the practice or after the meditation and before the yoga poses. You can decide according to the needs of your group. The other aspect of timing is duration. If you would like to recommend that the art practice be repeated daily then a simple, time-limited approach is best. Decisions about the length of time spent with art making depend on your perception of the group or individual's needs. Be sure that the complexity of the project matches the time you have allotted. Having a definite duration in mind before you begin is crucial. It will help the participants organize themselves and understand how to approach their creative work. Be sure to keep the participants appraised of the amount of time they have to complete the project, with reminders as the time winds down. Be aware that altering other aspects of the project will affect the timing as well, as you will see below.

Materials

In general, art therapists consider hard materials such as pencil, colored pencil, cut paper, etc. to be containing, or less likely than other materials to trigger an emotional response. Wet materials such as paint, watercolors or clay are recognized as more likely to evoke emotional reactions. Healthy individuals can regulate these influences easily. People who are stressed, or who have physical or mental conditions, may be more strikingly affected by the qualities of the materials. Notice the properties of the materials when you try out the project with a particular person in mind.

Size

The size of the project can vary according to the size of the paper or other material that is used, the intricacy of the approach or according to the amount of time allotted. Sometimes a small, simple project can be repeated to allow for a deeper understanding. Larger paper size could imply a longer duration for the project. Large paper may be difficult for some to tackle if they have little experience with art making.

Complexity

The project's complexity may be an issue for individuals who are intimidated by art making or lack confidence in their skills, or for those who have time limitations. A more complex project may appeal to an experienced practitioner, where meeting a challenge will serve to build personal strengths. For those less experienced try to break down the project into manageable pieces.

Experience level

No experience is necessary for any of the projects proposed in the yoga and art chart. As participants become more experienced with materials they can be offered more sophisticated materials and might be expected to attempt projects of greater complexity. However, complexity is not necessarily better. Working simply and quickly is often a strategy used to avoid the pitfalls of perfectionism, over-thinking and self-criticism. In many projects the complexity can be limited simply by reducing the time. Participants may find this kind of time limit freeing; they can release high or unrealistic standards knowing they only have a small amount of time.

Motor skills

Keep in mind your participants' level of motor skill. If grasping tools is difficult, pre-cut collage images can work well. In terms of precision, drawing materials are easier to handle than paint. Clay might be too difficult to manipulate for those with limited hand strength, but a softer three-dimensional material like Model Magic® could be ideal. Simpler projects of shorter duration might avoid frustration for those with motor skill difficulty; on the other hand, manipulating art materials is therapeutic for building fine motor skills. Be careful to offer breaks and maintain flexible expectations when presenting this type of challenge.

Considering clinical populations

By now you probably realize that yoga therapists recognize creativity as an integral therapeutic aspect of a yoga practice and that art therapists often acknowledge connections between yoga traditions and the use of art in a psychotherapeutic context. The purpose of this book is to envision the combination as a single endeavor, easily adapted to the needs of many different practitioners. Intention Centered Yoga and Art Therapy may be used appropriately with many different populations as long as it is mindfully adapted. The most important consideration is your familiarity with the population with which you are working. Your experience and intuition are the best guides. Some client populations requiring special consideration are children, elderly, inpatient, substance abuse, trauma, medical and hospice.

Children

Children, of course, have an affinity for creativity and have not yet acquired the restrictions of self-consciousness. For this reason, they tend to be open to experimenting with yoga and art. Accommodations may need to be made for limited attention spans and a tendency to become overstimulated. Some facilitators may prefer to begin the sequence of a session with children with art making, particularly if the group or individual is more culturally attuned to art making than practicing yoga. After focusing for a time on an art project they may be better able to attend to an intention meditation and then the session can finish playfully with yoga poses. Work with children should emphasize simple, direct explanations and shorter duration for each section of the practice, as compared with adults.

Elderly

Senior citizens vary widely in their activity levels, motor skills and cognitive functioning, so you will have to adjust the practice with sensitivity and perhaps offer choices. Chair variations can be offered for yoga poses and mudras can be simplified if necessary. The art offering can be adjusted as well according to the available facilities and the interest and abilities of the individuals and group members.

Inpatient

Working with inpatient groups in a psychiatric setting is a possibility. In this case it is helpful to keep instructions as concrete as possible for both yoga and art. Choices can be offered for variations of yoga poses. Keeping eyes softly open for meditation is a better choice for those who may become preoccupied with internal stimuli. The important consideration here is to be mindful of creating clear routines and using ongoing assessment to determine what yoga and art offerings are appropriate. Evaluate the potential practice in light of inpatient restrictions and regulations before implementing a particular practice.

Substance abuse

Yoga and art practice is well suited to this population as it is important to develop present moment awareness in order to be conscious of the strengths necessary to maintain sobriety. The emphasis on a focused intention is valuable for this group. Be prepared to relate the intention back to the overriding intention of sustaining sobriety.

Trauma

Those who have experienced trauma need special consideration. They might find it difficult to stay focused on body-oriented instructions. Inadvertent triggering can cause anxiety, dissociation and other defense mechanisms. Creating predictability and allowing for comfort with positions, movements and materials will help to create a safe environment. Those who have experienced sexual abuse might feel uncomfortable lying down on a yoga mat or being touched in any way. When working with trauma please offer choices, focus on the present and create routines, both in the yoga and the art making (Emerson and Hopper 2011).

Medical

Medical settings vary widely in their considerations and requirements. The key here will be to have a trusted medical professional who can advise about cautions and advantageous practices. Familiarize yourself with the symptoms and typical presentations of the medical concern. Work in a positive, supportive manner. Additional research may be necessary to work optimally. Learn what yoga poses and art materials may be contraindicated. Mudra and intention will be important with these populations. *Mudras for Healing and Transformation* by Joseph and Lillian LePage (2013) is a great resource.

Hospice

Clients in a hospice setting may be able to benefit from a modified yoga and art practice. Mindful breathing, mudras and intentions can be grounding and accessible and offer an opening for meaningful art making and discussion. Please remember to offer these practices to families and, if possible, to other caregivers.

Chapter 12

CONCLUSION

This book has grown out of a love and appreciation for the connections between yoga and art. Both yoga and art are activities that naturally promote mindfulness. The sense of being immersed in the present moment, necessary for both yoga practice and art making, begins a process of awareness, acceptance and healing. The guidance in this book is just one of many ways to combine yoga and art practices. Use of the Practice Chart (Table 5.1) in this book is flexible and graceful because at its center is the concept of intention. Intention begins when one imagines the solution to a concern. Allowing an intention to come into spoken form gives the practice momentum. The intention then informs all aspects of the combined practice.

The combination yoga and art therapy in the Intention Centered Yoga and Art Method was a response to my desire to design an approach that would have a wide application while providing attention to mind, body and spirit. First, it was important to have a convenient way to put the pieces together without reinventing the wheel each time. Creating a chart and having a handy reminder of the qualities of all the elements has made the process simple. The need for the chart grew out of my success with offering yoga and art therapy combined as a treatment modality.

I have used the chart for some time now in my art therapy practice and a number of advantages have become apparent. The physical grounding and repetition of therapeutic themes provide structure for those who are physically or emotionally ungrounded.

Beginning with yoga practices seems to enhance participant engagement while keeping defenses intact, and therefore provides a unifying experience which appears to allow greater ability to access emotional work. In groups I find that this method enhances group cohesion and improves consistency in attendance. Yoga and art therapy groups with consistent attendance seem to quickly develop a functioning and creative artistic identity and the clients become more intimately connected with their creative selves; art making flows naturally out of the relaxed and grounded state created by the group cohesion. Among the people I work with, crafting images from a place of calm stability seems to cultivate the ability to make changes at a deep level (Gibbons 2005).

Individuals and groups I work with often take note of personal differences and changes that have taken place over time, after participating in Intention Centered Yoga and Art Therapy. It would seem that the effects of awakening the body with mindful movement and awakening creativity through intentional awareness encourages engagement of inner and outer resources, so that the sum is greater than the parts. I am impressed again and again with this synergistic effect expressed in the quality of involvement from my clients and the genuine sincerity in their approach to art making.

I believe that the most notable commonality between yoga and art therapy is the mutual ability to give expression to the human spirit. I use this method in my personal practice as a way to address negative habits and to develop conscious positive intention for myself. I am always better prepared for life's challenges when my yoga and art practice is maintained. I also believe that personally and culturally we are at a disadvantage when we maintain separation of mind, body and spirit. The growth of our culture depends on cultivating a more holistic approach to relationships large and small; Intention Centered Yoga and Art is one small way to promote wholeness.

The heart of this book's information is held in the Practice Chart for Intention Centered Yoga and Art (Table 5.1). Practice the yoga and art together for yourself. Some effects will be subtle and some profound. Application of the sequences in the chart is open to your interpretation. As you develop your style and create space, intuitive discernment will guide you to find the approach that is both inviting and effective. Use this book as a guide to apply your knowledge, skills and creativity.

Intention Centered Yoga and Art Therapy is a method for those with an appreciation of both the power of engagement with art materials and the grace of yoga philosophy. Mingling art with yoga, mudra and meditation is seamless because ultimately they all connect you with your deepest self. They are endlessly variable and adaptive tools for giving form to intention. The beauty of this holistic approach is in its focus on benefits, solutions and positive change. The combination of modalities gives you and your clients many points of connection. However, healing, growth and change are not brought about by the application of a specific technique. Creating change depends on the individual, supported by relationship. Yoga and art together forge beautiful, productive bonds in the service of transformation.

REFERENCES

Preface

American Art Therapy Association (AATA) (2014) *About Art Therapy*. Alexandria, VA: American Art Therapy Association. Available at www.arttherapy.org, accessed on December 3, 2014.

Gibbons, K. (2013) *My Yoga and Art Adventure*. Brooklyn, NY: Karen Gibbons Yoga and Art NYC. Available at www.yogaandartnyc.com/my-yoga-and-art-adventure-in-which-i-have-several-sudden-realizations-and-some-slow-gaining-of-experience-leading-to-the-creation-of-yoga-and-art-nyc, accessed on December 3, 2014.

Kolter, S. (2014) "Flow states and creativity: The playing field." *Psychology Today, 2/25/14*. Available at www.psychologytoday.com/blog/the-playing-field/201402/flow-states-and-creativity, accessed on December 3, 2014.

LePage, J. and LePage, L. (2005) *Yoga Toolbox for Teachers and Students*. Sebastopol, CA: Integrative Yoga Therapy.

Introduction

Cope, S. (2000) *Yoga and the Quest for the True Self*. New York, NY: Bantam Books.

Diaz, A. (1999) "Brush with God: Creativity as Practice and Prayer." In T. P. Myers (ed.) *The Soul of Creativity: Insights into the Creative Process*. Novato, CA: New World Library.

Franklin, M. (2001) "The Yoga of Art and the Creative Process: Listening to the Divine." In M. Farrelley-Hansen (ed.) *Spirituality and Art Therapy: Living the Connection*. London: Jessica Kingsley Publishers.

Furman, L. (2013) *Ethics in Art Therapy: Challenging Topics for a Complex Modality*. London: Jessica Kingsley Publishers.

Goleman, D. (1995) *Emotional Intelligence*. New York, NY: Bantam Books.

Harvard Mental Health Newsletter (2009). "Yoga for anxiety and depression." *Harvard Mental Health Newsletter, 4/1/09.* Available at www.health. harvard.edu/mind-and-mood/Yoga-for-anxiety-and-depression, accessed on March 26, 2015.

Hass-Cohen, N. (2008) "Partnering of Art Therapy and Clinical Neuroscience." In R. Carr and N. Hass-Cohen (eds) *Art Therapy and Clinical Neuroscience.* London: Jessica Kingsley Publishers.

Kolter, S. (2014) "Flow states and creativity. The playing field." *Psychology Today, 2/25/14.* Available at www.psychologytoday.com/blog/the-playing-field/201402/flow-states-and-creativity, accessed on December 3, 2014.

Kraftsow, G. (1999) *Yoga for Wellness.* New York, NY: Penguin Putnam.

Malchiodi, C. A. (2006) *The Art Therapy Sourcebook.* New York, NY: McGraw Hill (originally published 1998).

Satchidananda, S. (2012) *The Yoga Sutras of Patanjali.* Buckingham, VA: Integral Yoga Publications (original work published in 1978).

Van der Kolk, B. A. (1994) "The body keeps the score: Memory and the evolving psychobiology of post-traumatic stress." *Harvard Review of Psychiatry 1,* 5, 253–265.

Weintraub, A. (2013) "The two way street: Integrating yoga into mental healthcare and mood management into yoga therapy." *Yoga Therapy Today: International Association of Yoga Therapists 9,* 3, 16–18.

Willitts, C. (2014) "Experience 'flow.'" *Mindful Strength.* Available at www. mindfulstrength.com/mindfulness-flow, accessed on December 3, 2014.

Chapter 1

American Art Therapy Association (2013) *What is Art Therapy?* Alexandria, VA: American Art Therapy Association. Available at www.arttherapy.org/upload/whatisarttherapy.pdf, accessed on December 3, 2014.

Art Therapy Credentials Board (2014) "Our mission." Greensboro, NC: Art Therapy Credentials Board. Available at www.atcb.org, accessed on December 3, 2014.

Bair, A. (2010) "Eight basic kinds of meditation (and why you should meditate on your heart." Institute for Applied Meditation. Available at www.iam-u. org/index.php/8-basic-kinds-of-meditation-and-why-you-should-meditate-on-your-heart, accessed on December 3, 2014.

Benson, H. and Klipper, M. Z. (2000) *The Relaxation Response.* New York, NY: Harper Torch (original work published in 1975).

Bhavanani, A. B. (2013) *Yoga Chikitsa: Application of Yoga as Therapy.* Puducherry, India: Dhivyananda Creations.

Cherry, K. (2014) "What is the autonomic nervous system?" *About Education.* Available at http://psychology.about.com/od/aindex/g/autonomic-nervous-system.htm, accessed on December 3, 2014.

Corliss, J. (2014) "Mindfulness meditation may ease anxiety, mental stress." *Harvard Health Publications, 1/8/14.* Available at www.health.harvard.edu/blog/mindfulness-meditation-may-ease-anxiety-mental-stress-201401086967, accessed on December 3, 2014.

Danhauer, S. C., Mihalko, S. L. and Levine, E. A. (2009) "Restorative yoga for women with breast cancer: Findings from a randomized pilot study." *Psycho-Oncology 18,* 4, 360–368.

Duch, W. (2007) "Creativity and the brain." *Cogprints, 5/2/11.* Available at http://cogprints.org/7300/1/06-Creativity-Brain.pdf, accessed on December 3, 2014.

IAYT (2014) "Learn about IAYT." Little Rock: International Association of Yoga Therapists. Available at www.iayt.org/?page=LearnAbout, accessed on December 3, 2014.

Kramer, E. (2001) *Art As Therapy: The Collected Papers.* London: Jessica Kingsley Publishers.

LePage, J. and LePage, L. (2013) *Mudras for Healing and Transformation.* Sebastopol, CA: Integrative Yoga Therapy.

McCall, T. (2007a) "Yoga therapy: Need to know." *Yoga Journal, 8/28/07.* Cruz Bay Publishing. Available at www.yogajournal.com/article/yoga-101/yoga-vs-yoga-therapy, accessed on January 1, 2015.

McCall, T. (2007b) "50 ways to heal a Yogi." *Yoga Journal, 11/18/13.* Cruz Bay Publishing. Available at www.drmccall.com/uploads/2/2/6/5/22658464/50ways.pdf, accessed January 1, 2015.

McDonald, A. (2010) "Using the relaxation response to reduce stress." *Harvard Health Publications, 11/10/10.* Available at www.health.harvard.edu/blog/using-the-relaxation-response-to-reduce-stress-20101110780, accessed on December 3, 2014.

Menen, R. (2010) *The Healing Power of Mudras: The Yoga of the Hands.* London: Singing Dragon (original work published in 2004).

Merriam-Webster (2014) "Meditate." *Merriam-Webster.* Available at www.merriam-webster.com/dictionary/meditate, accessed on December 3, 2014.

Rubin, J. A. (ed.) (2006) *Approaches to Art Therapy.* New York, NY: McGraw Hill (originally published 1998).

Stephens, A. (2009) "Relax – It's good for you". *Sydney Morning Herald,* August 20. Available at www.smh.com.au/lifestyle/relax--its-good-for-you-20090819-eqlo.html#ixzz1kQtHr9Pm, accessed on February 18, 2015.

Wallace, E. (1987) "Healing Through the Visual Arts: A Jungian Approach." In J. A. Rubin (ed.) *Approaches to Art Therapy.* New York, NY: Brunner/Mazel.

Yoga Alliance (2014) "What is yoga?" *Yoga Alliance.* Available at www.yogaalliance.org/Learn/About_Yoga/What_is_yoga, accessed on December 3, 2014.

Chapter 2

Davis, J. (2012) "The science of creative insight and yoga." Tracking Wonder. *Psychology Today,* 11/21/12. Available at www.psychologytoday.com/blog/tracking-wonder/201211/the-science-creative-insight-yoga, accessed on December 3, 2014.

Farhi, D. (2005) *Bringing Yoga to Life: The Everyday Practice of Enlightened Living.* New York, NY: Harper Collins (original work published in 2003).

Feen-Calligan, H. (2005) "Constructing professional identity in art therapy through service learning and practica." *Art Therapy: Journal of the American Art Therapy Association* 22, 3, 122–131.

Feen-Calligan, H. (2012) "Professional identity perceptions of dual-prepared art therapy graduates." *Art Therapy: Journal of the American Art Therapy Association* 29, 4, 150–157.

Franklin, M. (2001) "The Yoga of Art and the Creative Process: Listening to the Divine." In M. Farrelley-Hansen (ed.) *Spirituality and Art Therapy: Living the Connection.* London: Jessica Kingsley Publishers.

Furman, L. (2013) *Ethics in Art Therapy: Challenging Topics for a Complex Modality.* London: Jessica Kingsley Publishers.

Ganim, B. (1999) *Art and Healing: Using Expressive Art to Heal Your Body, Mind and Spirit.* New York, NY: Three Rivers Press.

Gregson, K. and Lane, R. C. (2000) "On the beginning of dyadic therapy: The frame and the therapeutic relationship." *Journal of Psychotherapy in Independent Practice* 1, 3, 31–41.

Hass-Cohen, N., Findlay, J. C., Carr, R. and Vanderlan, J. (2014). "'Check, change what you need to change and/or keep what you want': An art therapy neurobiological-based trauma protocol." *Art Therapy: Journal of the American Art Therapy Association* 31, 2, 69–78.

Iyengar, B. K. S. (1995) *Light on Yoga.* New York, NY: Schocken Books (original work published in 1966).

Julliard, K. N. and Van Den Heuvel, G. (1999) "Susanne K. Langer and the foundations of art therapy." *Art Therapy: Journal of the American Art Therapy Association* 16, 3, 112–120.

Lee, C. (2014) "Yoga 101: A beginner's guide to practice, meditation and the sutras." *Yoga Journal, 10/27/14.* Cruz Bay Publishing. Available at www.yogajournal.com/article/beginners/yoga-questions-answered, accessed on December 3, 2014.

Lusebrink, V. B. (2004) "Art therapy and the brain: An attempt to understand the underlying art expressions in therapy." *Art Therapy: Journal of the American Art Therapy Association 21*, 3, 125–135.

Malchiodi, C. A. (2006) *The Art Therapy Sourcebook.* New York, NY: McGraw Hill (originally published 1998).

Merriam-Webster (2014) "Holistic." *Merriam-Webster.* Available at www.merriam-webster.com/dictionary/holistic, accessed on December 3, 2014.

O'Conner, J. (2001) "Developing your intuition." *The Intuitive Connections Network. The Edgar Cayce Institute for Intuitive Studies, 11/26/08.* Available at www.intuitive-connections.net/issue3/oconnor.htm, accessed on December 3, 2014.

Plante, T. G. (2007) "Integrating spirituality and psychotherapy: Ethical issues and principals to consider." *Journal of Clinical Psychology 63*, 9, 891–902.

Ramm, A. (2005) "What is drawing? Bringing the art into art therapy." *International Journal of Art Therapy 10*, 2, 63–77.

Van der Kolk, B., McFarlane, A. C. and Weisaeth, L. (eds) (1996) *Traumatic Stress: The Effects of Overwhelming Experience on Mind, Body and Society.* New York, NY: The Guilford Press.

Chapter 3

DeBurijn, G., Kremers S. P. J., DeVet, E., DeNooijer, J., VanMechelen, W. and Brug, J. (2007). "Does habit strength moderate the intention-behavior relationship in the theory of planned behavior? The case of fruit consumption." *Psychology and Health 22*, 8, 899–916.

Downey, J. (2010) "Intuition series: How to create powerful intentions." *Very Smart Girls.* Available at http://verysmartgirls.com/manifesting/intention-series-how-to-create-powerful-intentions, accessed on December 3, 2014.

Dyer, W. W. (2010) *The Power of Intention: Learning to Co-create Your World Your Way.* Carlsbad, CA: Hay House (originally published 2004).

Gibbons, K. (2005) "Yoga and Art Therapy in Outpatient Substance Abuse Rehabilitation" (unpublished master's thesis). New York, NY: School of Visual Arts.

Grohol, J. M. (2005) "MIT explains why bad habits are hard to break." Psych Central. Available at http://psychcentral.com/blog/archives/2005/10/20/mit-explains-why-bad-habits-are-hard-to-break, accessed on December 3, 2014.

Satchidananda, S. S. (2012) *The Yoga Sutras of Patanjali.* Buckingham, VA: Integral Yoga Publications (first published 1978).

Chapter 4

Hass-Cohen, N., Findlay, J. C., Carr, R. and Vanderlan, J. (2014). "'Check, change what you need to change and/or keep what you want': An art therapy neurobiological-based trauma protocol." *Art Therapy: Journal of the American Art Therapy Association 31,* 2, 69–78.

Chapter 6

LePage, J. and LePage, L. (2013) *Mudras for Healing and Transformation.* Sebastopol, CA: Integrative Yoga Therapy.

McGonigal, K. (2008) "From hand to heart." *Yoga Journal, 8/1/08.* Cruz Bay Publishing. Available at www.yogajournal.com/article/practice-section/from-hand-to-heart, accessed on December 3, 2014.

Menen, R. (2010) *The Healing Power of Mudras: The Yoga of the Hands.* London: Singing Dragon (original work published in 2004).

Chapter 7

Allen, P. (2014) "Intention and Witness." In L. Rappaport (ed.) *Mindfulness and the Arts Therapies.* London: Jessica Kingsley Publishers.

Kabat-Zinn, J. (2005) *Wherever You Go, There You Are.* New York, NY: Hyperion (original work published in 1994).

McNiff, S. (2014) "The Role of Witnessing and Immersion in the Moment of Arts Therapy Experience." In L. Rappaport (ed.) *Mindfulness and the Arts Therapies.* London: Jessica Kingsley Publishers.

Rappaport, L. and Kalmanowitz, D. (2014) "Mindfulness, Psychotherapy, and the Arts Therapies." In L. Rappaport (ed.) *Mindfulness and the Arts Therapies.* London: Jessica Kingsley Publishers.

Chapter 8

Awaken (2013) "Quotes by Krishna Pattabhi Jois." *Awaken, 1/16/13*. Available at www.awaken.com/2013/01/quotes-by-krishna-pattabhi-jois, accessed on December 3, 2014.

Yoga Journal (2014) "Yoga poses." Cruz Bay Publishing. Available at www.yogajournal.com/category/poses, accessed on December 3, 2014.

Chapter 11

Dayton, T. (2000) *Trauma and Addiction: Ending the Cycle of Pain through Emotional Literacy*. Deerfield Beach, FL: Health Communications.

Emerson, D. and Hopper, E. (2011) *Overcoming Trauma through Yoga*. Berkeley, CA: North Atlantic Books.

Furman, L. (2013) *Ethics in Art Therapy: Challenging Topics for a Complex Modality*. London: Jessica Kingsley Publishers.

IAYT (2014) "Educational standards for the training of yoga therapists." Little Rock, AR: International Association of Yoga Therapists. Available at www.iayt.org/?page=AccredStds, accessed on December 3, 2014.

LePage, J. and LePage, L. (2013) *Mudras for Healing and Transformation*. Sebastopol, CA: Integrative Yoga Therapy.

Parker, S. (2013) "The use of touch in yoga teaching and therapy: Principles and guidelines for effective practice." *International Journal of Yoga Therapy 23*, 2, 69–70.

Weintraub, A. (2013) "The two way street: Integrating yoga into mental healthcare and mood management into yoga therapy." *Yoga Therapy Today: International Association of Yoga Therapists 9*, 3, 16–18.

Chapter 12

Gibbons, K. (2005) "Yoga and Art Therapy in Outpatient Substance Abuse Rehabilitation" (unpublished master's thesis). New York, NY: School of Visual Arts.

FURTHER READING

Allen, P. (1995) *Art Is a Way of Knowing.* Boston, MA: Shambhala Publications.

Allen, P. (2005) *Art Is a Spiritual Path.* Boston, MA: Shambhala Publications.

Darley, S. and Heath, W. (2007) *The Expressive Arts Activity Book.* London: Jessica Kingsley Publishers.

Desikachar, T. K. V. (1999) *The Heart of Yoga: Developing a Personal Practice.* Rochester, VT: Inner Traditions International.

Epstein, M. (2013) *Thoughts Without a Thinker.* Cambridge, MA: Basic Books (originally published 1995).

Forbes, B. (2011) *Yoga for Emotional Balance.* Boston, MA: Shambhala Publications.

Franklin, M., Farrelley-Hansen, M., Marek, B., Swan-Foster, N. and Wallingford, S. (2000) "Transpersonal art therapy education." *Art Therapy: Journal of the American Art Therapy Association 17*, 2, 101–110.

Judith, A. (2004) *Eastern Body, Western Mind.* Berkeley, CA: Celestial Arts (originally published 1996).

Judith, A. and Vega, S. (1993) *The Sevenfold Journey: Reclaiming Mind, Body and Spirit Through the Chakras.* Freedom, CA: The Crossing Press.

Khalsa, H. K. K. (2011) *Art and Yoga: Kundalini Awakening in Everyday Life.* Santa Cruz, NM: The Kundalini Research Institute.

Malchiodi, C. (2014) "Trauma-informed art therapy and trauma-informed expressive arts therapy." Available at www.cathymalchiodi.com/art-therapy-books/trauma-informed-art-therapy, accessed on December 3, 2014.

Radha, S. S. (2006) *Hatha Yoga: The Hidden Language: Symbols, Secrets, and Metaphor.* Spokane, WA: Timeless Books (originally published 2003).

Rama, S., Ballentine R. and Ajaya, S. (2010) *Yoga and Psychotherapy: The Evolution of Consciousness.* Honesdale, PA: Himalayan Institute Press (original work published in 1986).

Reis, J. (2014) "Mudras." Jennifer Reis Yoga. Available at http://jenniferreisyoga.com/resources/mudras, accessed on December 3, 2014.

Singleton, M. (2010) *Yoga Body.* New York, NY: Oxford University Press.

Stiles, M. (2002) "Yoga Therapy Center Joint Freeing Series." Crohns Forum. Available at www.crohnsforum.com/yoga/Joint-Freeing-Series.pdf, accessed on December 3, 2014.

Weintraub, A. (2003) *Yoga for Depression: A Compassionate Guide to Relieve Suffering Through Yoga.* New York, NY: Broadway Books.

Weintraub, A. (2012) *Yoga Skills for Therapists: Effective Practices for Mood Management.* New York, NY: W. W. Norton and Company.

Wiener, D. J. (ed.) (2001) *Beyond Talk Therapy.* Washington, DC: American Psychological Association (originally published in 1999).

INDEX